From Communism to Schizo
One man's long marc

To Emma,

Best wishes for
your future career,

Jeremy

From Communism to Schizophrenia and Beyond: One man's long march to recovery

Edited by
Gordon McManus & Dr Jerome Carson

With a foreword
by Professor Dinesh Bhugra CBE

Whiting & Birch
MMXII

© Whiting & Birch Ltd 2012
Published by Whiting & Birch Ltd,
Forest Hill, London SE23 3HZ

ISBN 9781861771209

Printed in England and the United States by Lightning Source

Contents

Dedications

For Gordon

This work is dedicated first and foremost to my mother, Gladys McManus, who has stood by me throughout my life through trial and tribulation. Secondly, the dedication also extends to my sisters and brothers, my nieces and nephews, grand nephews and nieces who have helped me in my illness. Thirdly, the book is also dedicated to the domino crew, Stanton, Karl, Keith and Simmo, who have made life meaningful despite my illness and special acknowledgements must go to Stanton and Eric Ayanlande Johnson.

Finally, this book is dedicated to those suffering from mental illness and who are trying to recover from its debilitating effects. I hope the contributions help in your recovery as they have helped me.

For Jerome

This book is dedicated to my Aunt Teresa and Aunt Bernadette. They are the only surviving siblings of my mother and father respectively. They have done more for me than words can ever acknowledge.

Notes on Contributors

Eric Ayalande Johnson is a poet, writer and historian.

Keith Bent is a qualified plumber and a fanatical Birmingham City Football Club supporter. He has been a friend of Gordon's for over a decade.

Dr Jonathan Bindman is a consultant psychiatrist with a community mental health team in Brixton. He is also clinical director for the Mood Anxiety and Personality Clinical Academic Group for the South London and Maudsley NHS Foundation Trust. He has worked in a variety of clinical settings, including Friern Barnet Hospital prior to its closure, as well as several community care services, including a home treatment team. From 1997 to 2005 he worked as a researcher at the Institute of Psychiatry.

Dr Jerome Carson was until August 2011 a consultant clinical psychologist in the National Health Service. He has now retired. He remains both interested in and involved with recovery initiatives.

Dr Peter Chadwick is a retired lecturer in abnormal psychology and personality at Birkbeck College, University of London. Following a psychotic episode in 1979 he has incorporated the experience into his research and teaching, producing many books, articles and broadcasts on psychosis. He believes in an integrative discourse of science, art and spirituality as the key to understanding and treatment in the field of psychosis.

Sophie Davies is a journalist who has written for Thomson Reuters, The Financial Times and The Independent on Sunday, among others. She is pursuing postgraduate studies in psychology and co-edited the recently published book, Mental Health Recovery Heroes Past and Present.

Stanton Delgado also known as 'DJ Stan da Man.' He has worked in the past as a mental health youth support worker.

Charlene DeVilliers has worked in Secondary Community Mental Health services since 1997. She currently manages Assessment and Treatment services in South Lambeth. Her first degree was in psychology, followed by a Masters in Social Work and a further Masters in Health and Social Care Management, and an Advanced Award in Social Work.

Gloria Giraud is Gordon's sister. She has recently retired and is a grandmother.

Dr Duncan Harding is an NIHR clinical lecturer and specialist registrar in forensic psychiatry, currently training in the South London and Maudsley NHS Foundation Trust. His research work is based at the institute of Psychiatry.

Dr Frank Holloway is an Emeritus Consultant Psychiatrist with the South London and Maudsley NHS Foundation Trust and former chair of the Rehabilitation and Social Psychiatry Faculty of the Royal College of Psychiatrists.

Daisy Masona is a Registered General Nurse, Registered Mental Nurse and Registered Midwife. She has worked in a various fields within health services holding managerial, teaching and research Posts in the National Health Service, community services and the private sector. Her passion is in mental health where she has concentrated her nursing career. She completed post graduate studies in Mental Health Management and hopes to complete her MBA Degree.

Gordon McManus is a former teacher, political activist and chess player.

Claudette Miller has worked in mental Health services for 28 years and was team leader for a Recovery and Support team until October 2011. She currently works with the Behavioural and Developmental Disorders Psychiatry Team and is studying for an MSc in Advanced Leadership.

Karl Miller obtained a degree from Essex University in Computer Studies in 1975. He has known Gordon for 38 years.

Dr Rachel Perkins worked for mental health services for 30 years and has been using them for 20 years. Formerly Director of Quality Assurance and User Experience at South West London Mental Health NHS Trust, Rachel is now chair of Equality 2025 - the cross Government Strategic Advisory Group on Disability issues – and works on the national Implementing recovery – Organisational Change (ImROC) programme.

Dr Glenn Roberts has recently retired from clinical; practice following 20 years as an NHS Consultant in Rehabilitation and Recovery in Devon but prefers to describe himself as, 'freelance' rather than 'retired.' He has greatly valued the creative struggle involved in writing and teaching as a support for exploration and understanding and continues to promote a cultural change towards person-centred and recovery-oriented approaches towards research and development projects and advisory roles with local, national and international organisations in the valued company of fellow travellers.

Dolly Sen is a writer film maker and artist. She has worked in mental health since 2001, including being one of the founders of Creative Routes, a Peer Trainer with the country's first Recovery College and a Development Worker for England's first Paranoia Groups Project. Her website is www. dollysen.com

Foreword

Schizophrenia is one of the most debilitating and devastating of diseases to be faced by patients, their carers and their families. Diagnostic patterns have changed over the past few decades; in the same period, therapeutic techniques and newer medications have also emerged, with increasingly great success. Yet no numbers of drug trials or therapeutic interventions can explore the individual patient's experience. The turmoil in their inner world, the symptoms and consequent behaviours are with the patient all the time. The therapist may see the patient for short periods on a regular basis, but patients and their families have to live with the illness the rest of the time. Therapists often tend to focus on the therapeutic hour and on symptom reduction rather than on symptom management. The patient perspective of their illness is critical in therapeutic engagement.

Recovery as a word and concept has become fashionable in the past decade. Yet different definitions exist in which the concept carries different meanings. Recovery is holistic and personal where the patient is able to manage symptoms and be socially active and functional. The individual patient's understanding of what recovery means to them and what it does is critical in creating a therapeutic expectation which can then be delivered in a pragmatic manner.

Therapist-patient interaction and relationship is at the core of therapeutic alliance and adherence. The patient comes to the therapeutic encounter with certain expectations. These depend upon their understanding of their distress and potential explanations which will be influenced by a number of factors. The therapist will see the patient with a certain viewpoint, depending upon their training and experience. Patients present with illness where their distress has taken on a social dimension, but clinicians may be interested only in disease, that is simply pathological aspects. This tension needs to be resolved if the therapy is to succeed. It is clear that Gordon and Jerome have managed to resolve this tension successfully, and this book emerges as a result of their therapeutic relationship. The book is unique in that it also allows other professionals who worked with Gordon to explore their journeys. The responses of friends and colleagues make this a moving and learning journey. This book offers a unique insight into many journeys – in tandem is the best way to describe this process. There is no doubt that patients learn much from their therapists, but I believe that we as therapists learn much more from our patients. We learn not only about their symptoms but, most importantly, about their inner world and how they manage and cope with their illness. The drive that Gordon shows is remarkable, but equally remarkable in this context are Jerome's skill and understanding, without any preconceived ideas or prejudices. This is what makes a therapeutic relationship work, where each side can be honest, open and caring. The therapist has to care as much about the patient and the patient must have faith in the therapist and the therapeutic strategy. This book offers a mirror to both patients and the therapists. More importantly, it should be read by carers and their families, who can then try to make sense of the patient's experiences and their inner world as well as feelings and behaviour. This book is a supreme example of working together to learn and to improve the lives of patients who are suffering from debilitating illnesses, and of those carers and families who suffer with the patient's turmoil. The focus on recovery is laudable. One of the major challenges in psychiatry is whether we have the outcome measures right and whether these measures focus on symptom reduction, symptom management or social functioning. Gordon and Jerome deserve our thanks for being open about their experiences and work and their faith in each other. There is plenty to share and learn here, and this book should be read by every mental health professional and trainee.

Dinesh Bhugra CBE
Professor of Mental Health & Cultural Diversity
Institute of Psychiatry, King's College London
President-Elect, World Psychiatric Association

Introduction

This book *From Communism to Schizophrenia and Beyond: One man's long march to recovery*, has been three years in the making. The idea for the book came out of sessions between the two of us. It is not of course the first time that a therapist and a patient have sat down to write a book together (for example, see Thomas and Hughes, 2008) and of course it will not be the last. This book originated from our joint quest to understand the new recovery approach, both in Jerome's desire to try and apply the principles of recovery to his clinical work and from Gordon's desire to try and recover himself, from schizophrenia. We start this chapter with short accounts from Gordon and Jerome as to why we wrote the book, we then provide a summary for the reader of the chapters that follow.

Why I decided to write this book? Gordon' story

The writing for this book did not come easy. When Dr Carson and I discussed it I hesitated. I was not sure that I could do it. Dr Carson had confidence in me, but for myself I did not want to think about it. He persuaded me and I agreed. In the latter part of 2008 he sent me two chapters for the book by Peter Chadwick and Dolly Sen. I had not done any writing on the subject matter at this stage. I was afraid to confront my mental illness, especially unpleasant memories of schizophrenia, and this was preventing me from writing even though I was still experiencing symptoms of schizophrenia. I was impressed by both chapters but it was Dolly's chapter that changed my attitude. Her chapter starts with the attempt to kill her father and how in the process of the attempt seeing a photograph of a young Dolly on the wall changed her life. For me it meant that Dolly had the resolve and determination to change the course of her life. This was inspiring. I said to myself 'if Dolly can write, I can do it'. I owe Dolly a great debt of gratitude for giving me the inspiration to write this book.

The second person who influenced me in the writing for this book is Dr Rachel Perkins who, in an article she wrote that I read in mid-2007, she said that 'you need hope to cope'. This 'saying' is part of my daily mantra in helping me to cope with the symptoms when they arise. The writing for this book was premised on her 'saying'.

The book is about coping with mental illness and trying to have a meaningful life and in this sense the service users' contributions have helped in my recovery stage. It is this factor that I would like the reader to bear in mind. Coping with mental illness is very difficult and there are many who have not coped and who have not recovered. This book is intended to give them some understanding of others who are coping, and have coped with mental illness. If you cannot cope you cannot engage in recovery. It is only when you cope with your mental illness that there can be a meaningful life.

Then there is Dr Roberts' own account of mental illness. Dr Roberts has stated elsewhere that 'Recovery is hard work'. It is hard work and Dr Roberts' chapter is an expression of perseverance.

My understanding of recovery is not only drawn from my experiences of the last twenty years from 1991 onwards, but also from Patricia Deegan, where she talks about 'attitude' and other factors that have helped her, and from Bill Anthony's and Retta Andresen's definitions. This 'philosophical basis' was expanded in the chapter by Drs Harding and Holloway. Thirty years ago I was very interested in Philosophy, especially materialist dialectics. During the years of 24/7 schizophrenia, from 1995 to 2003, I did not interest myself in this 'passion'. Drs Harding and Holloway 'awakened' this passion. The reader should pay serious attention to their discussion on the 'nomothetic' and 'idiographic' approaches to mental health treatment. For myself, I came away with the understanding that there should be dialectical interaction between the objectivity of medical science in mental health treatment and the subjectivity, e.g., stories and narratives, for example, of the mental health service user. Their chapter is an important contribution for the Recovery Movement in Britain. The 'idiographic' lags behind the 'nomothetic' and needs to catch up and this is the importance of their chapter.

For myself this book is not about me. It is not an autobiography even though I do talk in a limited sense about my life, but this is from the viewpoint of my mental illness – schizophrenia. This book, for me, is about Recovery and the Recovery Movement in Britain through the various contributions. Many of the contributors are service users and it is my privilege to be in the same book as them.

Finally, this book shows the 'hard work' that Dr Carson has done to ensure that service users engage in Recovery. His work or therapy with him has helped me to rationalise and bring logic to my illness, and his chapters' show that mental health medical practitioners should be 'on tap' not 'on top'. Even though Dr. Carson is aware of the' nomothetic' approach, he gave more emphasis to the 'idiographic' approach, of which we the service users are the beneficiaries. I am grateful to Dr Carson for his four and a half years of therapy. I have improved a lot even though I am not completely free of the symptoms of schizophrenia.

Why I decided to write this book? Jerome's story

The recovery approach brought me two main sources of excitement. First, it was obvious that the more I read about the topic of recovery, the more it became clear that there was no agreed recovery manual. Recovery is a very individual approach, though there are those who would 'manualise' it. Second, the recovery approach meant engaging with the people who use our services in a completely different way than we have ever done before. Gordon talks about mental health professionals being 'on tap, not on top.' This was of course one of the most important precepts to come out of the Sainsbury's Centre Report, 'Making Recovery a Reality,' (Shepherd et al, 2008). There are two experts in recovery. The first group are experts by their professional training. The second are experts by their personal experience of mental illness. Despite having worked with hundreds of people who have suffered with depression and psychosis, try as I might, I have no proper understanding of what it feels like to suffer with either of these conditions. Of course this makes mental health professionals who have experienced mental illness themselves uniquely placed to contribute to the debate on recovery. We have been fortunate in this book to have chapters from Peter Chadwick, Glenn Roberts and Rachel Perkins, all of whom have experienced mental health problems.

The recovery approach requires mental health professionals and the people who use our services, to work together in a different way. Gordon told me that he feels it may require services to undergo a complete paradigm shift in more conventional ways of working. Some writers have suggested that recovery work requires mental health professionals to adopt a 'coaching' role (Roberts and Wolfson, 2004). Personally, I feel a partnership model may be better for working with some individuals. Each of us comes with a different skills set into the therapeutic encounter. Michelle McNary had skills, knowledge and experience of film making. The project we decided on, of her making a film about recovery, which also featured Gordon, formed part of her own recovery. My role was to try and help Michelle obtain the resources to make the film, which with the help of Dr Frank Holloway and Dr Paul Wolfson, we succeeded in doing. Similarly Matt Ward the actor brought many talents from his background in acting. We were able to work together to put on the Conor McPherson play 'St.Nicholas,' which we used with the help of Yvonne Farquharson, to get across a positive message about recovery (Ward et al, 2010). So it was with Gordon. If Gordon had not become a scholar of recovery, there would have been no book. Readers will see from Chapter 2, that Gordon always wanted to be a communist revolutionary. Unfortunately, Gordon went from being a communist philosopher to suffering with schizophrenia. Now he is moving beyond schizophrenia to learn about and experience recovery. For Gordon it has been a long march, much longer than Chairman Mao's revolutionary march. For me, it has been a privilege to have walked with him for four and a half years of his journey thus far.

The Structure of the book

The book is in two parts. The first is concerned with Gordon's life and his own journey of recovery. It features contributions from the professionals who worked with him and also family and friends. The second half looks at roads to recovery. It features chapters from a number of recovery experts, several of whom have experienced mental illness themselves.

In **Chapter 1**, Gordon outlines his background. He talks about his interest in politics starting when he lived in Burma. Coming to England when he was 13, he then tells us about how he became interested in student politics, at secondary school, college and then at university. The bulk of the chapter is taken up with Gordon's involvement in British Communism. He talks about his connections with the different organisations that represented communism in Britain. He was also interested in international issues and became especially involved in the anti-Apartheid movement and the Irish Republican struggle. Having dedicated so much of his passion and time to the political struggle, it is hard not to feel sorry at the way he was treated by both individuals and organisations within the communist movement. As someone with a very strong grasp of communist philosophy, his theoretical contributions were at times undervalued.

At the age of 39, Gordon first began to experience serious mental health problems. These slowly deteriorated over a few years until he had his first hospital admission. A number of further admissions followed, four in total, two under a Section of the Mental Health Act. He was picked up on the street on one occasion after he waved a knife at a man in a car, who turned out to be a plain clothes police officer. Chapter 2, details his prolonged period of mental illness. For a couple of months after the death of his father, his 'voices' left him and he even started taking driving lessons. Sadly, the 'voices' returned, and he was admitted to hospital for the fourth and last time. Gordon eloquently refers to these years as his lost years.

In **Chapter 3**, Gordon talks about his journey of recovery. Informally, this really started when his sister gave him a computer, and he started playing chess against the computer programme. He also used the computer to start work on a study of globalisation. Another important factor was continuing to play dominoes with some old friends after his social club, The Studio, closed down. This maintained a level of sociality. In a formal sense, his recovery started when his consultant psychiatrist of the time, Dr Stephen McGowan, referred him to the PICuP Clinic at the Maudsley Hospital. This is a specialist service which offers cognitive behaviour therapy to individuals experiencing psychosis. Gordon completed a six month programme of therapy there. After this, Gordon's community psychiatric nurse, Simon Gent, suggested to him that he was probably suffering with 'post therapy depression,' and that he probably needed more therapy to get over this! Simon fortunately referred him to Jerome and their first session took place in January 2007. Together they developed a model of Gordon's illness and recovery, which formed the basis of a presentation to the South-West Sector Recovery Group (Morgan and Carson, 2009). This was attended by over 20 people, including both service users and staff. Gordon has gone on to give a number of other presentations about his illness and recovery, most notably to a group of over 40 social work masters students at Kingston University. While Gordon was previously a lecturer in business studies, he prefers to be interviewed by Jerome on these occasions, though in truth, Jerome does little of the work, other than asking the questions.

Chapter 4, presents the perspectives of the professionals who have worked with Gordon over the years. Charlene deVilliers was both Gordon's social worker and his care co-ordinator. She was also the person who had to instigate the process to have Gordon sectioned under the Mental Health Act. Gordon did not appreciate this at the time. Dr Jonathan Bindman was the consultant psychiatrist looking after Gordon then, and he talks about the problems in managing individuals with varying degrees of insight into their conditions. He also talks of the shock of seeing Gordon so unwell and hostile, and that it was hard to accept that this was the same individual who he got on with so well when he was mentally stable. Claudette Miller talks of her involvement with Gordon when she was with the case management service and the importance of medication concordance. Daisy Masona, sees in Gordon, a symbol of the hope that now prevails in psychiatry, after decades of disappointments. She feels the advent of atypical neuroleptic medications is transforming psychiatric care.

The dominoes crew are interviewed at the start of **Chapter 5**. Karl Miller and Gordon were at Essex University together and were flatmates for a while. Keith Bent and Stanton Delgado were friends from The Studio. Together the four of them meet once a fortnight in Gordon's flat to play dominoes and have a drink. Gordon provides the venue and also cooks them all a curry. Gordon is blessed to have such good friends and yet each of them in turn feels blessed to have known Gordon. The evening when we all sat down together was one of the most memorable occasions Jerome has ever had, and it was obvious to see and feel the love and affection which these men held for Gordon. Eric Ayalande Johnson, has known Gordon for 25 years, and has clear memories of Gordon since he was 10 years old. Eric has also seen Gordon at his most unwell. Despite Gordon's behaviour towards Eric when he was ill, this never deterred Eric, though he had no first-hand experience of major mental disorder till he met Gordon. The chapter ends with a tribute from Gordon's older sister Gloria.

In Chapter 6, Jerome shares his reflections of working with Gordon. The work with Gordon was especially important, as it was one of the first attempts Jerome made to try and put the recovery approach into practice. Apart from developing a model of Gordon's illness and recovery, Gordon also came up with a very short definition of recovery. It is that 'recovery is coping with your illness and having a meaningful life' (McManus et al, 2009). Jerome shared a lot of journal papers on recovery with Gordon, who in turn would go off and study them and come back and discuss how they related to his experiences. At times it was difficult to know who was the teacher and who was the student. They worked together for a four and a half year period and this book is a product of that collaboration.

Part 2 looks at different roads to recovery. In **Chapter 7**, Jerome takes us through the chronology of his own career in psychiatry. He explains a number of recovery based initiatives that he worked on in the Lambeth South-West Sector, some of which involved Gordon. One of the most successful of these was the recovery film, made by Michelle McNary. Gordon had no hesitation in agreeing to be a part of this film, despite the fact that people from across the globe would get to learn about his mental health problems. Jerome has also suggested, along with Gordon, that for the professional, recovery can also be hard work (Carson, 2011).

Chapters 8 and 9, feature two chapters written by Dr Peter Chadwick. Peter is someone whose work is well known to both Gordon and Jerome. No other individual has managed to write in so much depth about his experience of psychosis. He has brought unique insights from the fields of psychology, philosophy, literature, spirituality, art and biography, which have helped elucidate our understanding of psychosis. In the first of his two chapters he tells of how his background in Lancashire set the scene for his later developing a psychotic breakdown. Whilst in a psychotic state he threw himself in front of a London Route Master bus. Fortunately the driver's reflexes meant that he sustained comparatively minor injuries and the orthopaedic surgeons even managed to piece together his broken right hand in a way that he would still be able to hold a pen, as writing was so important to his livelihood. In his second chapter, he wonders if any good can come out of a psychotic episode? His own life is surely an affirmative answer to this question. He is not the only psychologist to have had a close encounter with death and come back to make a major contribution to the field (May, 2011).

Chapter 10, starts with the dramatic image of Dolly Sen standing over the sleeping body of her father with a knife in her hand poised to kill him! Fortunately she stopped herself and as she says, probably avoided being sent to Broadmoor. Elsewhere, I have described the conditions of her upbringing as Dickensian (Sen, 2011), and no doubt the trauma of her upbringing led to her developing psychosis at the very young age of 14. Dolly has long been a heroine of Gordon's and Jerome has run a number of recovery training events with her. At the time of writing her chapter, she was studying for her degree. Since then she has graduated with a first class honours degree and is working in the country's first ever Recovery College, as a trainer with lived experience. There are few better writers.

Chapter 11 sees Dr Duncan Harding and Dr Frank Holloway share their reflections as two psychiatrists on *Recovery*. They draw our attention to the distinction between nomothetic and idiographic approaches to recovery. They link the former to outcome studies and the latter to individual journeys and service user narrative. They see a need for a complete change in how psychiatrists work with their patients, towards developing more collaborative and empowering doctor patient relationships.

In **Chapter 12**, Dr Rachel Perkins describes her career as a clinical psychologist, mental health activist and more latterly as a service user herself. She has always held to the notion that work is the most empowering approach to recovery. Throughout her career she has battled to try and ensure that people with mental health problems had access to proper jobs, and not just therapeutic earnings.

Dr Glenn Roberts shares two main stories with us in **Chapter 13**. The first is a story taken from the history of medicine and concerns the centaur Chiron, the original wounded healer from Greek Mythology. The second is his own story, as both a psychiatrist and also a wounded healer himself. He has been one of the leading proponents of the importance of narrative, in a world that is increasingly dominated by evidence based medicine and the randomised controlled trial.

Finally, in **Chapter 14**, Gordon and Jerome reflect on the lessons they have learned from writing and editing the book. The book has covered virtually all the time they worked together, and indeed in his first session, Gordon reflected that maybe he ought to write a book. It was only a year later that they both began to seriously consider this possibility. It is our sincere hope that whether you are a sufferer, mental health professional, carer, friend or just someone who happened to pick up the book as it had an interesting title, that you discover as much hope and encouragement about the possibility of recovery from mental health problems as we have found in its pages.

Gordon McManus and Jerome Carson
London October 2011.

References

Carson, J. (2011) Recovery: the long and winding road that leads... In, Cordle, H. Fradgley, J. Carson, J. Holloway, F. & Richards, P. (Eds) *Psychosis Stories of Recovery and Hope.* London: Quay Books

May, R. (2011) Rufus May. In, Davies, S. Wakely, E. Morgan, S. & Carson, J. (Eds) *Mental Health Recovery Heroes Past and Present.* Brighton: Pavilion

McManus, G. Morgan, S. Fradgley, J. & Carson, J. (2009) Recovery heroes- a profile of Gordon McManus. *A Life in the Day,* 13, 4, 16-19

Morgan, S. & Carson, J. (2009) The Recovery Group: A service user and professional perspective. *Groupwork,* 19, 1, 26-39

Roberts, G. & Wolfson, P. (2004) The rediscovery of recovery: open to all? *Advances in Psychiatric Treatment,* 10, 37-49

Sen, D. (2011) Dolly Sen. In, Davies, S. Wakely, E. Morgan, S. & Carson, J. (Eds) *Mental Health Recovery Heroes Past and Present.* Brighton: Pavilion

Shepherd, G. Boardman, J. & Slade, M. (2008) *Making Recovery a Reality.* London: Sainsbury's Centre for Mental Health

Thomas, J. & Hughes, T. (2008) *The A-Z Guide to Good Mental Health: You don't have to be famous to have manic depression.* London: Penguin

Ward, M. Chander, A. Robinson, S. Farquharson, Y. & Carson, J. (2010) It's a one man show. *Mental Health Today,* 32-33.

Part One

One Man's Long March
to Recovery

I
Political Life

Gordon McManus

In this opening chapter, Gordon describes his early interest in politics, with his curiosity dating from when he was only 10 years of age in Burma. He then takes us through his involvement with school activism, leading to his developing radicalism at university. He felt that the university authorities wanted to exploit his knowledge of the Black community for dubious ends. Expressing his desire to enter revolutionary politics after he left university, his father's response was to show him the door! His decision to enter communist politics also alienated him from many of his friends. Gordon describes at length the 'battles' he went though in several communist organisations, with his acceptance, then later expulsion from these. One particular individual, K.N., proved to be a long standing collaborator, but they too eventually had a parting of the ways. Gordon also became involved in a number of major international issues, such as the anti-Apartheid movement, the Palestinian struggle and most particularly the Irish republican struggle for independence. Frustrated by years of his own personal study and struggle and political warfare, he eventually came to the decision to leave politics altogether. One of the talents he brought to this political work was his huge commitment and his detailed understanding of communist and socialist theory. British communism was said to be theory 'light.' Gordon's talent for theoretical understanding was to stand him in good stead later on in his life, when he began to understand and unravel the mysteries of recovery.

I first became politically conscious in 1962 when I was ten years of age. The military took over Burma and I started to read the newspapers to find out what the situation was. In 1963 the military steered the country onto a socialist-orientated path by nationalisation of foreign companies. I read this in the 'Working Peoples' Daily'. It was the first time I came across the concept 'Socialism'.

I came to England in 1964. In 1965 I went to Tulse Hill Comprehensive School. It was the first time I came into contact with the West Indian Community. Tulse Hill had a strong West Indian schoolboy population. I started to mix with West Indians and this was my first political act in this country. Forty three years ago Asians did not mix with West Indians and I had to break this prejudice which I did. In 1968 one of my friends became a Black Panther. His name was Linton Kwesi Johnson and I learnt from him about the struggle against racism not only in society but also within the school.

I, however, became political when I studied at Kingsway Further Education College, NW1. I, as an Asian, became one of the founder members of the first Black Student Society at Further Education level in 1972. I was elected Treasurer. This was the respect given to me as an Asian by Black students. There were those who did not see me as Black. An African girl came up to me and said that I was not Black which surprised me. In the political sense I saw myself as Black. This was the only time that I had any problems. I can now state that I carried out my duties in the service of the Black Student Society. It was an enjoyable period in my life.

In 1974, I went to study at the University of Essex. In my first year, I became Chairperson of the Third World (First) Society. During my tenure the Society had meetings on Palestine, South Africa and the Black struggle in this country. I was regarded as a 'radical' in my student days. This was noted by the University authorities.

In 1976, I suffered paranoia when I discovered that the University were watching me. The story goes like this. At the end of my final year at Essex 1976/77, I was regarded as a First/2.1 candidate for my degree. In October 1976 I was called in by the Linguistics Department to discuss my degree prospects. The lecturer pointed out that there would be difficulty with getting a First, because I had got a Third in one of my courses. All the students who sat that course got a Third, because during the examination one of the students had a breakdown and none of us could concentrate. The Linguistics Department refused to let us resit the exam. The Lecturer pointed out that a 2.1 was probable. He added a rider. The Department would recommend me for a scholarship to Georgetown University to do an MA in Sociolinguistics as long as I 'behaved' myself. I said I would think about it. A few weeks later, the Head of Department called me in. He said that the Department wanted me to do research on the language of domino games in the West Indian Community and to give the conclusions to the police. I refused and changed my research project. This was the first time I came across the State in the representation of the Linguistics Department. They had been watching me, a 'radical' student, reading the Georgetown Journal of Sociolinguistics for my research project. This was why I was surprised at the 'recommendation'. I was heavily affected by this act of the staff of the Linguistics Department. I left disillusioned and angry with the University after completing my degree. Suffice to say I did not come out with a 'good degree'.

After completing my studies I stayed at my parents' home for a year. In 1978 my late father spoke to me and said that 'Gordon, if you want to be a revolutionary, get out of the house'. I left home and shared a flat with a University friend who I am still friends with today. That friendship has lasted thirty-four years even through my illness.

For the next two years I studied Scientific Socialism because I had decided to become a Communist, which I was drawn to at University. I read and studied 'Das Kapital' and other works by Marx, Engels and Lenin. I made my speciality dialectical materialism, based on the economics of Marx.

The decision to be a revolutionary communist was not supported by my family and friends. They positively encouraged me not to get involved with Communist politics. I felt a bit lonely and dispirited.

In 1980 a Communist whom I knew well, K.N., came back to Britain after living in the Soviet Union for about a year and a half and decided to join the New Communist Party (NCP). He asked me if I wanted to join the NCP. I decided to give it a go even though I favoured the Communist Party of Great Britain (CPGB).

The history of these two organisations in the late 1970s set the context. In the 1970s divisions arose within the CPGB between the 'Eurocommunists' and the hardline Stalinists. In 1977, the Stalinists broke away from the CPGB and formed the NCP. I was against this breakaway as it did not help the cause. Unity was more important than any breakaway party that was formed. In my view this division was detrimental to the Communist cause for the next twenty five years. The touchstone for being a communist was whether one was 'Pro-Soviet'. I had my doubts over Soviet socialism because of the domination of the State, but I did not have any alternative clear ideas. I, nevertheless, at that time, saw that being 'Pro-Soviet' was important in developing Scientific Socialism, flawed as Soviet socialism was.

The main task that I set myself was to connect the Black Struggle for Equality and Justice and against racism with the Left.

I joined the NCP by becoming a member of the Wandsworth Branch. The leadership of the NCP, which included the General Secretary and the Editor of its paper, the New Worker, were some of the members of this Branch. At the first meeting that I attended with K.N., we were categorised after the meeting as 'intellectuals' by the General Secretary. He said 'Let's see what they are made of'. Such was the mistrust that developed from the start. We were also subject to a probationary period of membership.

This compounded the 'mistrust'. The NCP was a small organisation and it needed new younger members. The 'mistrust' was also due to an inner-party struggle with young communists in the NCP with some being expelled. All I knew was that I had to act in an exemplary and comradely way to obtain full membership after the probationary period.

I got involved in Branch activities. These included selling the Party paper, the New Worker, engaging in the peace movement, working in your Trade Union and the local Trades Council, and participating in studies within the Branch and political discussions. At this time I also got interested in the Irish struggle. K.N. and I got involved in the South London Hunger Strike Action Committee. The Branch did not want us to get mixed up in this as it was run by the 'Ultra-Left' – the Revolutionary Communist Group (RCG). The NCP however was not active in the Irish Hunger Strike of 1980-81. It was the time of Bobby Sands and the other hunger strikers and support had to be given in the face of Mrs Thatcher's, the British Prime Minister's stubbornness. The struggle for Irish unification was not headed by the mainstream Communist organisations, the CPGB and the NCP. It was led by what was regarded as the 'Ultra-Left'. This caused tensions with the NCP leadership because they did not want to be tainted with 'Ultra-Leftism' and to a certain extent K.N. and I were regarded as a bit 'Ultra-Leftist'.

For the NCP, the peace movement was the major issue, not Ireland and its unification. It was important to fight for the Irish National struggle, as Engels pointed out that a country which oppresses another cannot be free. Twenty eight years ago, British Imperialism still dominated the Six Counties. Britain could not be freed as long as it was oppressing the Irish through partition. This was not understood by the mainstream communist organisations, the CPGB and the NCP in **practice**. As the great German idealist philosopher Hegel remarked in his moment of realism or materialism, that 'practice is a criterion of truth'. The practice of the NCP on the Irish question was non-existent and was only words not deeds. K.N. and I tried to make up for this deficiency.

The political work that I engaged in on Ireland during this period, taught me a lot about Communist practice. It was dominated by 'Marxism-Leninism' developed by the Communists of the Soviet Union. The book that the branch decided to study during this period was called the 'Battle of Ideas' (Communist Party of Great Britain, 1958). It expressed the ideological differences between 'Marxism-Leninism' and bourgeois ideology. The issue was which was the scientific ideology, and 'Marxism-Leninism' laid claim to be the dominant scientific ideology? This book taught me a lot at that time about the dominant ideology of the International Communist movement, that is, 'Marxism-Leninism'. I knew that NCP members were regarded as 'tankies' (allusion concerning Hungary and Czechoslovakia) or Stalinists, but I was more concerned with developing Scientific Socialism.

When our probationary period came to an end, there was a branch meeting in which K.N. and I were excluded. The Branch members discussed our full membership in secret. It was not an open and democratic discussion about our full membership. I was very disappointed with the approach of Wandsworth Branch of the NCP. It later became clear that they acted on the orders of the NCP leadership, especially the General Secretary, which also had its HQ in Wandsworth. They called us in eventually and said that we were accepted as full members.

It did not mean that we could 'relax' as they were still 'suspicious'. I got 'engaged' in polemics with an NCP member who worked at Party HQ. Westacott had just written an article in the Party's journal, the New Communist Review, on unemployment. He gave a presentation to the Branch. I disagreed with him because he had confused and conflated the relation between unemployment in the transition from feudalism to capitalism with the 'industrial reserve army' (Marx) in a mature capitalist economy. He said to reply to him in the journal which I did. It took me a month to write the reply, as his article was a mess. I did the bulk of the writing even though there was collaboration between K.N. and I. He wrote the beginning which dealt with Lenin's principle of 'professional revolutionaries'. The Editor, who was the General Secretary, edited out this section by K.N. even though I ensured that the reply was under our joint names. The General Secretary offered me a 'post' on the Party paper and I suggested to him that K.N. should also work on the paper. He disagreed and I refused. I felt that both of us working on the Party paper would have enhanced its quality, especially as K.N. had experience in this field in the Soviet Union.

It was around this period that K.N. started to propagate Lenin's principles of 'professional revolutionaries' and a 'paper aimed at the level of the advanced workers'. I supported him after I had done my own research through reading Lenin. There now took place a 'battle' between K.N., supported by myself, with the NCP Branch and national leadership. Branch meetings became tense and friction was developing between the protagonists. It was a difficult period. K.N. said that the majority of Branch members supported the Party leadership, which was to be expected. There were times when 'comradeship' went out of the window. I did not expect such behaviour. I was new to the British Communist movement and I had not been involved in battles over Lenin's principles before. This 'political situation' was new to me. K.N. was aiming for the NCP to be a 'Leninist party'. He wanted the NCP to be a 'vanguard Party'. The NCP leadership, I think, also wanted the NCP to be a 'vanguard Party' but the question was: Did it want the NCP to be a Party of 'professional revolutionaries' with a paper aimed at the level of the advanced workers? This was where the NCP leadership disagreed with K.N. and me.

It is important to understand the approach of K.N. to understand subsequent events. Whilst K.N. was conducting an important 'inner-party struggle' within the Wandsworth Branch, he extended it to the Southampton Branch. His ex-girlfriend was a prominent member of the Southampton Branch. He contacted her and persuaded her to propagate the concepts of 'professional revolutionaries' and ' a paper aimed at the level of the advanced workers.' That Branch came to accept these principles and put a resolution to the 1981 Party Congress after a struggle. I did not want to factionalise and I told K.N. about the situation. I argued that we should establish ourselves in the NCP first, before coming out with full frontal assault on the Party leadership. This should be done at the 1983 Congress. He disagreed. He said that he would be expelled by then, so he wanted the 'war' to be at the 1981 Congress. I stayed away from this factionalism, but became 'tainted' with it. I carried on with Branch work, for example, selling the Party paper. There were the unemployment demonstrations of 1980-81. K.N. decided to go up North (Liverpool) to get support for Lenin's principles, but it was the demonstration that surprised me. First of all it was the first time I had been to the North of England. Secondly, it was the biggest demonstration and the first of many demonstrations that I attended. Only the anti-Apartheid demonstrations later in the 1980s came close. I began to understand working class politics. It was not a revolutionary situation but these unemployment demonstrations were expressions of working class politics in Britain.

K.N. and I had been in the NCP for nearly a year before matters came to a head. It was the 1981 Party Congress held in London. Southampton Branch put in a resolution, which everyone knew had the imprint of K.N.. The resolution was defeated and the General Secretary stated that he would take 'administrative measures' which meant expulsions. K.N. was expelled together with members of the Southampton Branch. Two members of the Wandsworth Branch resigned in protest. Members of the Southampton Branch resigned as well. I did not resign and this caused friction between K.N. and me. I wanted to carry on the struggle to 1983 and vowed to fight on. I was not immediately expelled. The NCP leadership, which was essentially the General Secretary, decided that I should have a discussion with the new Editor of the New Worker, the Party Paper, to retract my support for a 'paper aimed at the level of the advanced worker'. His arguments were so low level that I refused. He reported back to the General Secretary and the Party leadership and I was expelled.

I suffered from a strange catharsis. I was shocked that having joined a communist organisation, I would be expelled within a year. I felt that my communist 'life' had come to an early end.

The period with the NCP was a new and bewildering situation. The struggle for the implementation of Lenin's principles brought out strange reactions. It is my view that the Party leadership, following the General Secretary, was incorrect to act in such a harsh manner. If there were any controversies, then expel those involved, was the policy of the NCP leadership. They may have viewed the situation as 'acting in the interests of Imperialism'. The behaviour of Communists was seen as either acting 'objectively in the interests of Imperialism' or 'subjectively in the interests of Imperialism'. The NCP felt that developing Lenin's principles was not in the interests of the Party.

After we were expelled we met to discuss what to do. I was finished with the NCP but K.N. and A.F. from Southampton wanted to carry on fighting for reinstatement. Together with P. and T. from the Wandsworth Branch, who resigned in protest, the decision was eventually made to write a critical analysis of the NCP leadership's position.

The international political situation was tense. There was Poland and Solidarity. Poland raised the question of whether socialism was under threat. There was the situation of Afghanistan's move towards communism. There was Saddam Hussein and the war with Iran and his persecution of Iraqi Communists. There was the Reagan-Thatcher axis which confronted socialism and the Soviet Union. The Cold War was at its highest in intensity. There was the Irish Struggle. There were difficulties and differences within the CPGB with the 'Eurocommunists' in the ascendancy.

The critique of the NCP by K.N. was called 'Economism, Tailism and the New Communist Party'. During this period K.N. had to keep together the small group that had formed from the fall-out in the NCP. They decided to call themselves Proletarian. K.N. spoke to me that there were difficulties in Southampton and would I help out. I decided to do so and went down to Southampton on a Sunday in 1982. I proposed that K.N. chair the meeting and that we have structure as the group was 'loose' in structure. It was agreed. T. came down but not P. who was a Black worker - one of the few black workers in the NCP. Twenty eight years ago there were not many Black Communists and most of them were in the CPGB. The most well known was W.P, who was a member of the Central Committee of the CPGB and whom I first met in the early 1970s when I was active in the Black Student Society at Kingsway College. I disagreed with him in the early 1970s over being a communist but here in 1982 I was involved in communist politics.

I agreed with K.N.'s analysis of the NCP, but I had my own view about that organisation. The British communist movement suffered from 'Economism' and 'Tailism' but in the case of the NCP it was, in my view, 'Workerist' and failed to act on Lenin's principles. My experience in the NCP showed me that organisation was incapable of acting as a vanguard party. The leadership of the NCP in 1981 lacked theory. Engels made this criticism of the English in the nineteenth century and this was still the case in the second half of the twentieth century within the British communist movement. The politics of the NCP was concerned with attracting the popular masses and the working class in particular, but its failure to comprehend theory especially Lenin's principles, meant that in reality, in practice, this organisation would be at the periphery of working class politics. As Lenin pointed out to the International Working Class that: 'Without revolutionary theory, there is no revolutionary movement'. The object for myself was that I would be guided by this principle as a communist. I was concerned with the development of theory and its application to social practice, that is, communist practice. During this period I had been researching the British neo-Althusserians, who represented the Eurocommunists in the CPGB. I came to the conclusion that they were 'neo-Kantians' and not materialist dialecticians. Hindess and Hirst came to the conclusion of rejecting Scientific Socialism. I had been noting the development of their work since studying them at Essex University and I was not surprised at their conclusion. They tried to turn Marx upside down though 'criticism' and their rejection of Scientific Socialism failed.

However, the basic division in the British Communist Movement was between those who were 'Pro-Soviet' and those who were 'Eurocommunists'. I decided to join Proletarian. I was quickly regarded as a 'senior' figure even though there were differences between K.N. and myself. The first Organising Committee (OC) consisted of K.N., A.F. and myself. We, as an organisation or group of Communists, decided to carry on working on the Irish Question especially on the Hunger Strikes and the consequential political activities that arose.

I was the first National Organiser of Proletarian but I did not do a good job. It was because, first of all, Proletarian was not a national organisation with national membership. There was only Southampton and London. It was difficult to develop national activities when your membership base was limited. For example, meetings could not be arranged in the North because

Proletarian did not have members there.

I was moved to education and because of my 'theoretical understanding,' especially Marx's *Capital*, I was able to develop a course. Proletarian began with studying Illyenkov 'Dialectical Logic,' which was at that time my 'bible,' as it gave you a good introduction to Marx's *Capital* (Illyenkov, 1977). The second work of 'Marxism-Leninism' that Proletarian studied was again Illyenkov's 'The Abstract and the Concrete in Marx's Capital' (Illyenkov, 1982). I have to state now that these works by Illyenkov were some of the best produced by Soviet 'Marxism-Leninism'. There were other works that were studied. They ranged from Lenin's 'Materialism and Empirio-Criticism' (Lenin, 1996), to standard Soviet works on Political Economy – Capitalism and Socialism. When Proletarian developed a Central Committee at K.N.'s suggestion, I became responsible for Education. I give credit to Proletarian members because they did their best to come to terms with 'theory'. In my view and from my experience in the British Communist Movement, the British Communists are poor at 'theory'. That is what makes them 'lag' in British politics.

There was also study of K.N.'s work 'Economism and Tailism within the New Communist Party'. Southampton with A.F. in the lead, was given the task of writing a definitive work on the Irish Question. They found it a difficult task. A.F., in particular had difficulty with dialectics, even though she was doing a PhD at Southampton University. It was decided that K.N. would take over the task. It took him about a year and a half to get to grips with the subject matter and he managed to get to grips with dialectics and began to understand 'real contradictions' and its relation to the Irish situation. He did a good job even though his marriage was coming under strain. Proletarian had to educate itself because it was propagating the concept of 'professional revolutionaries' and 'paper aimed at the level of the advanced workers'.

At the beginning of Proletarian's development I was privy to K.N.'s views, but he still had 'distrust' over the situation in the NCP concerning myself. As Proletarian developed over the next four years, there was distancing between K.N. and myself. I was privy to his understanding of communist development because I had known him and A.F. since 1974. I knew he was a communist and pro-Soviet and pro-Leninist. He came from a working class background and it was this that drove 'his politics'. His room at Essex University accommodation was full of Lenin's works. A.F. came from a middle class background. It was said to me that her father was a Professor in English. I however did not care about their class background as long as they developed socialist theory concerning Britain.

The article was finished in 1984 and K.N. did a good job. It was at that time the best written by a communist organisation in Britain. There was a discussion over the title. I suggested 'Proletarian Internationalism and the Irish National Question' which took into account both the national and the international. After much discussion it was accepted. The problem arose with the Editorial which was an affirmation of Pro-Sovietism in an absolute sense. In this sense, I had my doubts. I had not done a study of the Soviet Union and its history but I was still pro-Soviet. The Editorial argued that the Communist Party of the Soviet Union (CPSU) was a 'principled Marxist-Leninist Party'. The subsequent events of the late 1980s were proof that this position was erroneous.

K.N.'s work became priority studying material for Proletarian members and those who wanted to know about the communist position on Ireland. It was the product of four years of activity on Ireland by those who were NCP and Proletarian members.

I got to know the British Left and members of international communist organisations who were political refugees in Britain during my time with Proletarian. In Britain, there were four principal trends within the British Left and they were the Communists, the Trotskyites, the Maoists and the anarchists. There were those who began to distance themselves from Trotskyism, like the Revolutionary Communist Group (RCG), which was welcomed even though they were not fully pro-Soviet. I learnt a lot from the RCG and their supporters. They were slightly mistrusted as to their role on the Irish Question and 'Ultra-Leftist'. Their policy on Ireland was more important than the considerations of the Irish people. This was the problem with the RCG. When K.N. wrote Proletarian No.2 on the Irish National Question there was criticism of the RCG at my instigation. One of their late leaders said that 'Dialectics is mumbo jumbo' (I think, even though I was there when he said it) and Proletarian should criticise them for being 'anti-theory'. The RCG took umbrage. When Proletarian No.2 came out, members of Proletarian sold it including myself at a major demonstration in the morning. The RCG brought a few copies so as to ascertain the 'criticism' against them. They were seething but we were not attacked. I spoke to K.N. and told him nothing happened at the demonstration. In the afternoon there was a meeting which was attended by K.N., A.F., and N. but they were physically attacked by the RCG. Such thuggery did not serve the RCG well. I was disgusted by the behaviour of the RCG. The British Left has to develop through 'criticism and self-criticism' and polemics not through physical attacks when they disliked something. That is for fascist groups. I was not attacked even though they knew I was in the leadership of

Proletarian. The reason was because I was Asian/Black (in political terms of those days). It would have made the RCG look foolish. In my view, the RCG was not guided by revolutionary theory and this made them veer towards 'Ultra-Leftism' but I would say in their favour that their members and supporters showed that they were committed.

The work that I did on Ireland for Proletarian brought me into contact with Irish people. I got to know the relatives of the Guildford Four. I met G.M. who was a highly respected Irish political activist who had spent nearly two years in a British Prison on false charges. I met him and his partner, V. later and got to know them well. He was a major force in trying to unite the Irish political activists because Sinn Fein in Britain was breaking up. Our working relationship was 'professional'. I got to know him through working on the Irish Political Prisoners campaign where he was the convenor. I represented Proletarian and through our work he showed, at least, respect for Proletarian. We put our money where our mouth was through giving a donation for the campaign. However I got to know him personally and met his father and brothers. I thank him for educating me in the Irish people's struggle for freedom and unity. I also met John McCluskey who spent ten years in prison (six years in solitary confinement). I met his wife later at the Sinn Fein Congress in Dublin for a brief introduction.

I got to understand Irish revolutionary culture. I used to go to Irish pubs to hear Irish revolutionary songs by Irish bands. My favourite was 'The Boys of the Old Brigade'.

I got to understand that the Irish were the first people to be colonised by the English and they were very conscious of this fact. Before Black people suffered racism there was prejudice against the Irish.

The most important event in the brief history of Proletarian was commemoration of the 40th anniversary of Soviet troops entering Berlin in 1985. We were in discussion with a Soviet representative who was the Pravda Correspondent. It was initially envisaged that there would be a 'Unity' meeting with the NCP and the CPGB on the subject, but they did not want to be involved. I was given responsibility of 'technical matters', for example, microphone and speakers, but I did not do a good job and K.N. got very angry as he regarded it as a failure. The meeting was held at the Marx Memorial Library with a Soviet representative called Bogdanov. It was for K.N. and members of Proletarian the recognition by the Communist Party of the Soviet Union (CPSU) that Proletarian were a legitimate communist organisation within the British Communist Movement. K.N. reminded me of this constantly and it was his highest achievement as a 'Pro-Soviet' Communist. I had my doubts. For me, Proletarian had to pass the 'test of time'. It had a long way to go before it became a 'vanguard party'. It takes years to develop scientific communist leadership. Proletarian had only being in existence for three years and I felt that matters were being handled in 'haste'. The struggle affected personal relationships and K.N.'s marriage came under strain. During this time the Central Committee decided on K.N.'s proposal to 'give their lives to the struggle'. It was to show solidarity with the communist cause. A political bureau had been formed with K.N., A.F. and N. as full members (in effect, the leadership of the organisation) and I as 'alternate member'. I was not privy to any discussions on relations with the contingents of the International Communist Movement.

In 1986 I was asked to stop work on Ireland and work on the Anti-Apartheid issue. I got involved with Lambeth Anti-Apartheid Group. Proletarian (London) had decided to work on South Africa. The three major national liberation struggles in the 1980s were the Palestinian Struggle, the Anti-Apartheid Struggle and the Irish National Question. The African National Congress (ANC) and the Palestinian Liberation Organisation (PLO) were regarded by Margaret Thatcher, the then British Prime Minister, as 'terrorist organisations'. Now over twenty years later, the ANC is the government of South Africa, the PLO, the government of the Palestinian territory and Sinn Fein is developing a peaceful path to the 'unity of the Island of Ireland' through full participation in bourgeois democracy in the Six Counties, where it is engaged in 'power-sharing' with the Democratic Unionist Party (DUP).

I became Vice-Chair of Lambeth Anti-Apartheid Group (LAAG) and attempted to develop Proletarian's policy within the local Group. There were problems with the City Group – a front of the RCG – which had to be resolved. There was the reorganisation of the Anti-Apartheid Movement in London based on the Borough system. Lambeth had to be developed. The Chair, who was a white South African, did not attend committee meetings regularly due to other commitments and this was affecting LAAG. I decided that there was a need for a new Chair and recommended that I become the Chair which was accepted by the LAAG committee. I developed a plan that LAAG should have links in the community – the local trade unions, the Black Community and religious organisations and local political organisations, like the Labour Party. It was once this objective was reached that Proletarian's policy could be implemented as LAAG would have the support of the representatives of the community. I got involved with M.M., a black South African, who I thought was a member of the ANC, who was trying to develop Lambeth Council's Anti-Apartheid policy. I remember that he showed me an ANC calendar of events. The next meeting we had, he said that the Pan-African Congress (PAC) and the Black Conscious representatives had developed their own calendar and did I 'leak' it to them. I said 'No'. I was surprised that I could be viewed like that. To this day, I do not have knowledge of who was responsible. It was through M.M.'s instigation that I became involved with the ANC. He advised me to see the late M.D. Naidoo at the ANC Office in North London to discuss matters of local issues with the ANC. The local 'Ultra Left' in Lambeth was up to all kinds of things on the Anti-Apartheid issue and the ANC wanted to be kept abreast of matters. It was M.D. Naidoo who asked me to work 'secretly' for the ANC. He wanted me not to tell anyone and I was to report to him on any matters affecting LAAG. I told him that what I would be doing would come into conflict with Proletarian but he said not to worry. I decided that my internationalist duty was more important than working in Proletarian. It was also the case that one does not turn down an opportunity to work with a national liberation organisation when asked. During this period I was removed from Proletarian's Political and Central Committees and was reduced to an ordinary member at K.N.'s decision. K.N. said that it was in the 'revolutionary interest'. I was surprised. I spoke to M.D. about it, but he told me to work in the Anti-Apartheid Movement. I also spoke to him about calling him at the Office from my home. He got upset over that because he thought that my phone would be tapped. I did not know how to conduct 'secret work'. All I was doing was reporting to him on Anti-Apartheid issues in Lambeth. Proletarian with K.N. at the helm, decided that I should no longer be Chair and decided to remove me with their influence on the LAAG committee. I spoke to M.M. about it and he said that I should speak to M.D. I went to the ANC Office but the door was shut on me. I never went back, I left politics altogether.

During the early period of anti-apartheid work I came across black organisations that I made connections with for Proletarian, for organisation to organisation discussions. I spoke to K.N. about it and letters of invitation were given. It was the Political Committee with K.N. and A.F. who entered the discussions on behalf of Proletarian. At a meeting with one black organisation there were problems with A.F. who acted in a heavy-handed way. K.N. spoke to me and included me in the next round of discussions with this black organisation. The meeting went well and there were no problems with A.F. I was surprised that I was not included at all the meetings with these black organisations, as I was the leading black member in Proletarian. I felt at that time that problems were surfacing with my political relations in Proletarian

A few months later, the former LAAG Chair came to see me and told me that my name was in disrepute and he said that I should rejoin LAAG to clear my name. I agreed with him.

K.N. came to see me and told me that the Central Committee had made the wrong decision and that I would be reinstated to my former position. I told him that unless the Political Committee was 'Liquidated' I would not be rejoining. He said 'No' and I did not rejoin Proletarian.

Looking back on this period I went through a strange situation. This situation brought about paranoia and problems in wanting to know who or whom to trust in political activity. I trusted the ANC representatives but there were doubts in me as to whether they trusted me, given my limited experience on the Anti-Apartheid issue. I knew that the ANC was a genuine national liberation organisation and working for them was no problem. The problem was with Proletarian.

In the late 1980s – around 1989 I became more paranoid and decided to see what Proletarian was doing with an intention to rejoin. I found out that there were divisions within the Political Committee between K.N. on the one side and A.F. and N. on the other side. It led to the breakdown of Proletarian. That was my last contact with Communists and the Communist Movement, as I decided not get involved anymore. For eight years my life was fully engaged in political activity. I gave my all in terms of politics to the Irish patriots and people. I enjoyed this period of political activity and it was straightforward. I gave my all for the national liberation of the South African people, but it was a complex situation in Lambeth. All I can say is that I have never acted 'objectively' or 'subjectively' in the interest of Imperialism.

I stopped Anti-Apartheid activity in 1991 with the release of Nelson Mandela.

Reflections on the period 1980-87

It was an intense period for me who had decided to put the 'revolutionary interest' first before personal interests. I did not find that balance between the personal and the revolutionary. This period was the first time I had worked with 'white activists'. I learned a lot. In Proletarian there were heated discussions and controversies which I am not going to go into. All I can say is that I thank Proletarian members for contributing to my understanding of Scientific Socialism especially T. who attended a lot of meetings of importance with me. I apologise to R.B. and others over my attitude in certain situations in the early days of Proletarian.

The British communist movement was not united in the 1980s. There was no 'unity in action'. It was the major focus of the activities of the State because at that time 'World Socialism' led by the Soviet Union and the CPSU was a major power in world politics. Soviet recognition was important in order to develop relations with contingents of the International Communist Movement and to prove your credentials. This was the Proletarian approach. For me, 'revolutionary deeds' were important in being recognised as a vanguard force.

My views on Communism in 2008

The implosion of Soviet socialism and the disintegration of the CPSU was a heavy blow for 'Marxism-Leninism' and the International Communist Movement. I would briefly like to explain the situation.

The system of socialism that existed in the Soviet Union from Stalin to Gorbachev was the 'state-monopoly system' (Lenin). Lenin wanted Soviet Russia to embark on the path of developing socialism on the basis of the cooperative system. He argued that the 'system of civilised co-operators' was the system of socialism. In this relation, 'civilised co-operators' was an expression of socialist relations of production. With the development of the 'state-monopoly system' there was an 'absence of socialist relations of production' in the Soviet Union as the late Joe Slovo, the leader of the South African Communist Party pointed out. It meant that the workers living under socialism became alienated from the means of production because of state ownership. Lenin stated that, and I paraphrase him, theoretically speaking, state monopoly is not the best system from the viewpoint of socialism.

Marx, and he is followed by Lenin, argued that the cooperative system is the system of socialism. I agree with these great revolutionaries. I disagree with 'Marxism-Leninism' that the state plays a critical role in socialist economic development.

In the 1980s 'Pro-Sovietism' blinded communism from engaging in a debate on the system of socialism until Gorbachev came along. It was Gorbachev who recognised that the state monopoly system of socialism in the Soviet Union was leading to stagnation in the economy and problems for socialism. The majority of Soviet 'Marxist-Leninists' disagreed with Gorbachev and his 'faction' in the CPSU and these differences lead to the disintegration of the CPSU and to the implosion of socialism in the Soviet

Union.

I have come to another conclusion. Lenin argued that 'Imperialism is the highest stage of capitalism' (Lenin, 1996). This is the position that twenty first century 'Marxism-Leninism' holds fast. It is in my view incorrect. The developments within mature capitalism have led to great changes. The first point to note is that Lenin premised Imperialism on 'concentration of production and capital.' Concentration is one aspect of the General Law of Capitalist Accumulation discovered by Marx – the other three are: centralisation (capitalist expropriating capitalist), organic composition of capital and the industrial reserve army. This where Lenin 'differed' with Marx when he defined mature capitalism as Imperialism based on 'concentration'. Marx argued that in mature capitalism there would be the full application of the General Law of Capitalist Accumulation through its four aspects.

Modern mature twenty first century capitalism sees the full application of the General Law of Capitalist Accumulation. Centralisation not concentration has come to the fore. Centralisation takes the forms of 'takeovers', 'mergers', 'acquisitions' and so on which are expressions of capitalist expropriating capitalist and are fast becoming the major force in capitalist economic development. This was not the case in Lenin's time. What has superseded Imperialism? Globalisation has superseded Imperialism as the new higher stage of capitalism. Globalisation is the integration of the global capitalist economy based on the domination of finance capital and premised on the full application of the General Law of Capitalist Accumulation with centralisation being the determining aspect.

The third aspect of my difference with Marxism-Leninism' is concerned with Marx's concept of 'social humanity'. This is the 'standpoint' of the new materialism that Marx developed. 'Marxism-Leninism' has not developed this concept of Marx. For myself, Marx's concept of 'social humanity' has to be developed into 'socialist humanity'. The philosophy of Scientific Socialism is the philosophy of 'socialist humanity'. The reasoning is thus: 'social humanity' has to be transformed into 'socialist humanity' in the transition period from capitalism to socialism. It means that in relation to the economy there is propagated the cooperative system as the system of socialism, because the social ownership of the means of production results in the worker no longer being alienated or estranged from the means of production. The worker is the owner of the means of production and is at one with it. Under capitalism the worker is estranged from the means of production because it is the capitalist who owns the means of production not the worker. As regards the 'humanity' aspect it is that the individual is able and free to develop his faculties and interests. There is the propagation of universal human values common to mankind. It is premised on socialist morality and socialist values as a means of developing the creative abilities of individuals and families. The philosophy of socialist humanity has to be developed for the working class to grasp that link in the change that leads to the transition to socialism.

These are my major differences with 'Marxism-Leninism'. I have come to these positions in the period 2006 to 2008. This clarity of my communist thought has enabled me to recover and cope with the 'voices.'

References

Communist Party of Great Britain (1958) *The Battle of Ideas: Six Speeches on the Centenary of the Communist Manifesto* London: Communist Party.

Illyenkov, E. (1977) *Dialectical Logic: Essays on History and Logic.* Moscow: Progress Publishers

Illyenkov, E. (1982) *The Dialectics of the Abstract and the Concrete in Marx's Capital.* Moscow: Progress Publishers.

Lenin, V. (1996) *Imperialism, the Highest State of Capitalism.* London: Junius/ Pluto Press

2

From 1991:
The Years of Schizophrenia

Gordon McManus

The onset of schizophrenia began insidiously for Gordon in 1991. He believed that the Soviets were communicating with him, through a new science of 'mental telepathy.' It was not until 1994 that he became so unwell that he had to be sectioned and brought into hospital involuntarily. After his discharge he was put into Bed and Breakfast accommodation, until the council managed to find him a small flat. In October 1995, Gordon admitted himself to hospital, as he could not cope with the 'voices.' Due to his difficulty in dealing with the 'voices,' Gordon started self-harming, to show the 'voices' he meant business. This Gordon feels was part of his descent into madness and irrationality. Gordon hid the true extent of his illness from his family and friends, as well as from mental health professionals. Amazingly he was discharged from mental health services in 1999. The following year, all his benefits were stopped, and he had no gas or electricity in his flat. When out in the street one day, he threatened a man in a car with a knife. It turned out to be a plain clothes policeman and he was arrested. After spending a night in Brixton Prison, he was once more admitted to mental hospital. When he was discharged on this occasion, he faced possible eviction from his flat. His social worker and psychiatrist managed to help him avoid this and to get his benefits reinstated. For Gordon, these were part of his 'lost years,' the years of florid schizophrenia.

I stopped being a communist activist in the late 1980s after my problems with the African National Congress (ANC) and Proletarian. I maintained relations with the Lambeth Anti-Apartheid Group (LAAG) and was a member until the release of Nelson Mandela and the collapse of Soviet socialism. Proletarian policy had failed whilst I was absent from political activity within LAAG and the Group was developing the policy that I had developed before, which was basically the national Anti-Apartheid Movement policy. I was proved correct in my understanding of what LAAG policy should be.

It was in 1991, around May, that I had my first experience of schizophrenia. I was doing freelance lecturing in business studies. I was not on drugs. One evening I heard 'whispering' and I thought it was the Soviets trying to contact me through 'mental communication' because I had given my life to the communist cause. I did not think that I was experiencing mental health problems. I was absolutely sure that the Soviets had contacted me. The 'whispering voices' said to me to burn my books as I did not need them. I was unsure about this. However in the night I decided to burn some papers in the waste bin. I nearly set fire to the place I was living in and I decided to stop. I went to bed. The next day I told my landlord that I would like to burn my books and he agreed that I could do it in the back garden. I did not tell him why. It took me five hours to burn the books and journals that I had. A few days later I heard the 'voices.' These 'voices' were loud and they were abusive. I was surprised because it is rare for me to use abusive language. I thought the neighbours were swearing at me and I got very angry. These 'abusive voices' lasted about an hour. Eventually, the 'voices' left me and I decided to concentrate on my invigilation duties as it was the exam period at the college where I worked. The 'voices' stayed away until 1993, but I remembered this experience and decided to 'get even' with the Soviets who had affected my life. I was waiting for the 'voices' to communicate with me again. I was sure that the Soviets were going to contact me through 'mental telepathy'. I gave up teaching because of these 'voices' because I wanted to teach the communists responsible for affecting my life like this. I was going to use their methods to 'get even'. This was the delusion that I lived with for ten years – up to 2001.

In 1993, I was sharing a flat with my brother in Streatham, South London when the 'voices' returned. It was around October 1993. The first incident was of hearing a party next door. 'Voices' were coming from next door but most of them were abusive, which shook me. I checked through the window to see whether there was a party but the flat was dark. I was under the delusion that the Soviets were able to use the brain for their purposes and vowed to fight them. It was around this time that Karl came to see me to go to a poetry reading by Linton and others at the South Bank. I went with him and all during the poetry reading I heard 'abusive voices'. I managed to keep myself together till we got to The Studio in Brixton, when I suffered from nausea and Karl took me home. The nausea was due to fact that I was not eating well and should not have been drinking.

During this period the 'voices' were starting to become 24/7. It was constant and would not leave me alone. Another incident was when a girl I had fallen in love with at University - her name was L.R. - her 'voice' spoke to me in the most endearing terms. I was surprised. It made me feel that the 'voices' were being controlled by the Soviets.

I started to do some research on the implosion of Soviet socialism to prove to the 'voices' that I was highly developed in socialism. I discovered that the system was the 'state-monopoly system'. I also started writing 'A Reply to Joe Slovo's' pamphlet, 'Has Socialism Failed?' to prove my credentials to the Soviet and communist 'voices.' I borrowed my niece Jennifer's computer, and put on computer what I had hand-written. The voices started telling me what to delete and to use 'comrade' when addressing communists as I had the habit of using surnames only. This got me angry with the 'voices'. I did not view these 'voices' as schizophrenic delusions but the ability of the Soviets to control thoughts.

One of my brothers spoke to my parents and just before Christmas they decided that I should spend this period with them because he said that I was ill. I was taken to my parent's home and my mother and father looked after me. I was still under the 'delusion' that the Communists had found a new means of doing political work and that these 'voices' were from leaders of communist organisations, who were finding out whether I was 'fit' for the new method of communist work. In this sense, I was of the 'mind' that Joe Slovo, leader of the South African Communist Party (SACP) was communicating with me. Physically I was eating well again through my mother's care. The severity of my illness could be seen through the constipation that I suffered from for a few weeks. I would like to say that on the four occasions that I have been hospitalised I have suffered with constipation. This was the physical side of my illness.

In January 1994, I felt fit enough to return to Streatham. My parents had their doubts and so did my brother, but he agreed to have me back. For the next few months things were not so bad even though I suffered my first bout of sexual impotence. I thought the Soviets were trying to control my physical life and 'rebuild' it.

Comment

I kept this a secret until 2007, when I read James Bellamy's account of his schizophrenia (Bellamy, 2000). His was a truthful and honest account of his illness. It inspired me in 2007 to write about my problems. I wrote a short piece for Dr Carson. I was surprised that I experienced symptoms that were similar to James Bellamy. It was the first time I had written anything on my illness.

*

It was FA Cup Final day in May 1994 that my symptoms resurfaced with a vengeance. The day began in silence. I went to the barbers to have a haircut. I returned to my bedroom to watch the Final. As I was watching it two 'voices' of friends of mine from University days, who were Manchester United supporters, started talking to me. From then on the 'voices' came back. By late July, early August my condition became severe. I was very angry with the communists and was heavily paranoid. I carried a knife in my bedroom and started chopping the staircase. I even started to set my bedroom on fire then realised I would be in trouble and doused the flames. My brother realised that I was in a bad shape and went to Lewin Road for advice. Someone came to see me, but I refused to let them in. They came back again, this time with the Police. They broke down the door and arrested and sectioned me. I was taken to the South-Western Hospital and kept in a secure ward. I spent approximately three months in hospital and came out in late November 1994. I hid my condition from the doctors but they diagnosed me as having 'paranoid psychosis,' as they could not diagnose my condition accurately without my help.

When I came out I went to see my family but they accused me of things concerning my brother, which I do not want to go into, and which meant 'sour' relations with my family. I had no home to go to because my Landlord had me evicted due to my behaviour, so Lambeth Council put me into Bed and Breakfast accommodation. After a few weeks the Council found me a one bedroom bed-sit accommodation. I went to see my friend Karl and explained my situation. I told him that I had been in hospital. He took it casually. We played chess and after it I left. I went to see Linton and he asked me if I could help out in his office for the Christmas period. I did not want to let him down so I said 'Yes'. It kept me busy with something to do and kept the 'voices' at bay.

It was then that Linton's son, Eric and I, formed the beginning of our friendship. I had known him since he was a baby, but he was now grown up and I had not seen him for a few years. He asked me to teach him chess. I decided to use this as a means of keeping in touch with life. I also encouraged Eric with his poetry writing.

I finished working at Linton's office in late January 2005. I was offered a council flat in mid-January, which I accepted. At least I was stable and had a place I could call home. I have lived at this place from 1995 up to the present.

The 'voices' came back in February 1995. I was suffering from dental pain one day in late February. This went on for a few hours and the 'voices' became increasingly shrill as the hours passed. In the end the 'voices' told me, with spite, that one of my brothers was responsible for this pain. I try not to be a spiteful person and I was shocked at the way the 'voices' spoke to me. I swore to get even.

In April 1995 I was 'teaching' Eric chess but whilst I was doing this one evening, the 'voices' kept talking to me continuously and I had great difficulty keeping my concentration. It was the most difficult time. The 'voices' were keeping me awake at night and I had difficulty sleeping. Financially I was living on the bread-line.

In October, I could not cope with the 'voices'. I was occasionally seeing a communist in Brixton. I did not know whether he was still a member of the NCP, but he and I had an argument in 1981 and I remembered him. He was the brother of A.F., a Proletarian member. I felt like killing him every time I saw him. I went to Lewin Road to speak to the doctor about the 'voices'. He said to use a walkman to drown out the 'voices,' but it did not work. I went back to see him and told him that I would like to put myself in hospital voluntarily to help me control the 'voices'. I stayed in hospital for a few weeks and when I left I felt better. In November, Linton asked me whether I would help out in his Office for the Christmas period. I agreed and this kept me busy and distracted me from the 'voices'.

In January 1996, I suffered from back problems which meant that I could not walk for a few weeks. It was in 1996 that the 'voices' took a political form. I was trying to make sense of the 'voices'. I started to tell the 'voices' which side of my bedroom they could speak from. I began to structure the 'voices'. It was to try and use some logic and control the 'voices'. I put the ANC in one part of the room, the SACP members in another part, and the Labour Party representatives in another part of my room. In this way I tried to make sense of the 'voices'. I started to see 'forms.' At first it was headings from books that I had read. I knew that I did not have a photographic memory so I was surprised. I was under the 'delusion' that I did not need books and the Soviets with their 'forms' would educate me in a new way. I started to 'talk' to the 'voices' about dialectics as a philosophy. I even got out Hegel's 'Science of Logic' and discussed certain chapters with the 'voices' (Hegel, 1969). The only thing was that the 'voices' did not discuss Hegel with me but just talked about what they wanted which annoyed me.

It was around the middle of 1996 that I started to self-harm. I told the 'voices' that I would 'take my blood' in order to show them that I meant business. I used a Stanley knife to cut my hand. I was lucky that I did not sever a vein.

Linton came to see me and I told him about the Soviets and that I showed him the scars of cutting myself. He could not believe me and even asked a friend's wife who studied in the Soviet Union and she expressed the view that the Soviets had not developed such a science of mental communication. I even showed him my scars from self harming. I think he must have thought that I was suffering from a few 'loose screws'.

Comment

This was the descent into irrationality, the descent into madness. It lasted through the late 1990s. It was only in 2001 when Dr Bindman diagnosed me with paranoid schizophrenia, when I told him that I heard 'voices' that I realised that I suffered from a mental illness. During the late 1990s I hid my condition from the doctors and others.

•

The period 1996 to 1997 was occupied fully with the 'voices' and the 'forms'. I developed two different personalities. One was my individual personality which during the day I would 'talk' to the 'voices,' and a social personality when I went out in the evenings to The Studio. This was how I managed to hide my illness from people and friends. I managed to keep my 'delusions' quiet and even hid them from Eric who came to see me regularly during this period. On one occasion I got a knife and started saying to Eric that I was not afraid of the Soviets and would get them. He got a bit worried as he saw it as being out of character and that I might try to knife him.

In 1998 I decided to 'blank' Eric and Karl. They regularly attended The Studio. I 'blanked' them by cutting off all links with them because of the 'voices'. I used to sit in The Studio on my own and ignore them completely whilst mentally communicating with the 'voices'. It was around this period that I started challenging the 'voices' to come and see me in The Studio physically. No one from the political 'voices' turned up. All I was hearing was 'voices' in The Studio.

There was a strange thing that occurred during this period. I was sitting in my front room around 8pm when the voice of the partner of a friend of mine started 'speaking' to me. I was surprised because I had no interest in her in any manner whatsoever. 'She' started to express endearments that shook me. I said to her that I was not interested but the 'voice' kept on and on. It was like having a conversation with another human being except in this case it was a 'voice'. It lasted about 45 minutes and I was glad when it was over.

Another 'schizophrenic' situation was watching a football match whilst talking to the 'voices.' The 'voices' became abusive. I was angry at Zidane, the famous French footballer, because he was playing at the time. I asked the 'voices' whether Zidane was responsible for the abuse. The 'voices' kept on abusing me and I was very angry with the Soviets for subjecting me to such abuse. I swore to get even.

Around 1999, Dr Boocock became my psychiatrist. I hid my condition from her. I saw her regularly after she came to visit me at my flat in Brixton. My condition of hearing 'voices' was becoming very severe. The 'voices' and 'forms were becoming incessant. However, I did not want Dr Boocock to know my delusion, my secret, so to speak. Dr Boocock thought me well enough to discharge me. I did not know what I was doing. I was not fit to work. This is an objective assessment. I could not get a job and I was not in a fit state to work. My income support was withdrawn and housing benefits stopped. My brother gave me money but it was not enough to live on.

It was around this time that I got to know Stanton in The Studio. He had a 'quick manner'. In my bedroom I would see a quick form and I classified it as Stanton. I did not tell Stanton about it at the time. (I only told him in 2008).

During this period a woman I knew from The Studio asked me if I would help her out with her Diploma. She knew that I used to be a teacher and sought my help. C.W. wanted me to help her in her Diploma in 'Black Mental Health Counselling'. Here I was suffering from hearing 'voices' and I was trying to 'teach' a friend. At the first session I told the 'voices' not to disturb me, as I do not like any interference when I teach. I gave C.W. a crash course in essay writing and then started to explain to her what the topic was about. She got herself a computer to aid her in her course work. The peculiar thing was that the 'voices' kept going and there was a form associated with it, whilst I was 'teaching'. I warned the forms to be quiet but it did not happen. I had great difficulty concentrating for the next few weeks due to the 'voices' but I managed to help her with most of her course work. Towards the end I told her she was becoming too reliant on me and she needed to take a more 'independent' approach. We had a big argument and I left her flat. I did not speak to her for the next two years in The Studio. It was only in 2001, when I came out of the South-Western Hospital and I decided to renew my friendships, that I decided to speak to her again. I asked her in 2001 whether she passed her Diploma. She said 'yes'. I was pleased for her.

In 2000, the year of the Olympics, the 'voices' became very severe. They kept coming at fast speeds. My head felt like it was charged with electricity. The 'forms' were appearing with increasing regularity. I would watch TV for a while just to take a rest. I would return to my bedroom and there I would see the 'forms' of political people. There were 'forms' of George W Bush because that year was the US Presidential elections. I would get 'forms' of Milosevic, the Serbian leader and Saddam Hussein, the Iraqi dictator.

I 'ordered' their executions because of the genocide that they committed. I would get 'forms' of former Soviet leaders and I expressed to the 'forms' my views on socialism. I even got 'forms' of Blair and Brown who were the leaders of the British Government. I spoke to them by saying that they should manage capitalism first and then engage in the transition to socialism. Such were my 'delusions'.

I started to carry a knife everywhere. It was not because I was afraid. It was due to the fact that the 'voices' were affecting me. I even went to The Studio carrying a knife. and showed it to Simmo and he went and told C. C. told me that knife carrying in The Studio was not tolerated and he threatened to ban me. I told him I would cease carrying a knife in The Studio which I did, as I did not want any trouble with C. However, in my daily life I still carried a knife. I would go to The Studio and 'blank' everyone by sitting by myself unless someone joined me. I was left alone in The Studio. All I did while I sat and drank beer was to 'mentally' communicate with the 'voices.' I even played a game of Chess with S and the 'voices' were 'talking' to me while I was playing. I remember this because I lost a game that I should not have lost. I was regarded as the most advanced chess player at The Studio even before my illness. Whilst playing this game the 'voices' were saying to me that Karpov, the former world chess champion, was coming to The Studio. It was while I was waiting for Karpov to arrive that I lost concentration and resigned the game. Karpov, suffice to say, did not turn up. I was annoyed with the Soviets who had caused me mental anguish.

During the year 2000, my income support was stopped, and my housing benefit was stopped. I had no electricity or gas. The winter was approaching and it was getting cold. The 'voices' and 'forms' were intense.

One morning in early October, I think, I was going somewhere and I was carrying a large kitchen knife and also a Stanley knife. I was crossing the main road, Brixton Hill, to catch the bus when a car with three or four men in it came close to me. I took out my Stanley knife and flashed it at the car while finishing crossing the road to the bus stop. The next thing I knew was that the car turned around and one man came out and said he was a policeman and searched me and found that I was carrying out a knife. I was taken to Brixton Police Station arrested and charged with possession of knives. I told the Police that I was a mentally ill patient and the Police Doctor came to see the next day after spending the night there. I said he should speak to Dr Boocock. He phoned but she had other commitments and the Police Doctor did not do anything. The Police could not find a Magistrate's Court to try my case and I spent the next night in Brixton Prison. The 'voices' were afflicting me heavily. The morning after spending the night in Brixton Prison I was taken to court. In the prison van the 'voices' kept telling me that Linton was to be Prime Minister and I could not believe it. I said to the 'voices' that I wished Linton 'Good Luck'. The duty solicitor took my case on. She decided that I was unwell and pleaded to the Court to send me to hospital. The Magistrate agreed with her and I was taken to the South-Western Hospital by the Court psychiatrist. I spent about three months in hospital. Dr Bindman became my consultant psychiatrist. I think I was sectioned by the Court because I was not allowed to leave the ward as I was under the jurisdiction of the Law. In January 2001, I attended Court when I was a bit better. The Duty Solicitor informed the Prosecution that I was still in hospital and recovering and would they drop the charges against me. The Duty Solicitor, who was a woman, told me that the Prosecution agreed and that I was free to go. I returned to Hospital because I had not been discharged by Dr Bindman. I had not told Dr Bindman that I was hearing 'voices'. I still tried to keep my 'secret'. It was at the end of my treatment in hospital whilst I was in the process of being discharged when Dr Bindman told me that he had difficulty diagnosing my condition. I told him that I heard 'voices'. He diagnosed me as paranoid schizophrenic. I was a bit shocked.

Comment

I would like to thank the duty solicitor. To this day I do not know her name but I am very grateful for her care. I would also like to thank Dr Bindman and the nursing staff for the care and consideration they gave me in relation to my court case. They took great care of me.

*

When I came out of hospital I resolved to rebuild my life after my carer, my sister Laura, had spoken to me about schizophrenia. I had another problem. This was to fight the eviction from my flat by Lambeth Council. I had to go to the County Court. It was a letter from Dr Bindman that stopped the eviction order and persuaded the Judge. I was pleased. Charlene deVilliers became my social worker. She filled out my income support form. I could not even fill a form on my own. She also got help for me to redecorate the flat. I thank her and Dr Bindman for their care.

I returned to The Studio in March 2001, where I decided to renew my friendships with Eric, Karl, C.W. and others. It was during this period that I told Eric that I suffered from paranoid schizophrenia and he took it well. He kept the friendship. I beat him at chess and I said I would help him to improve. In December that year Karl came and asked me about Globalisation and the Marxist-Leninist understanding. I said to him 'Globalisation is Imperialism' and found out later through research of the South African Communist Party position that I was correct. I decided to do some research on the subject matter.

It was in the latter part of 2001 that I learnt that my father was dying from terminal cancer. I was affected by it. I even told Keith that this was the case and I also told him that I was suffering from 'depression'. I was still hiding my illness from my other friends. Keith only got to find out in 2007. My father passed away in May 2002. During this period the symptoms were still there, but they were not that severe. I could cope. It was after my father's death that matters took a strange course. From July 2002 to mid-September 2002 I was free of the 'voices'. I was surprised. I felt that I had overcome my grief for my father. I felt that I had recovered. I started doing driving lessons and hoped to then get a job. Unfortunately for me in September 2002 I broke down when the 'voices' returned.

One evening in September 2002, I walked into my front room and sat down. As I looked out of the corner of my eye I saw a blue form. I turned round and a 'voice' started to speak to me. I pleaded with the 'voice' to go away. I was no longer living the 'delusion' of Soviet mental communication. I knew it was schizophrenia. After this the 'voices' started to overwhelm me. They were incessant. I could not control it. I could not even engage in driving lessons. One day, as usual, I decided to do my driving lesson despite hearing 'voices'. The driving instructor realised that I was not well because my driving was erratic and drove me home. I have not taken driving lessons again. I stopped answering my phone. My sister, Laura thought it strange and because she had a spare key decided to visit me. I wondered who was entering the flat. It was my sister. I threw her out. She spoke to Dr Bindman and Charlene. They came to visit me and advised me to enter Hospital. I refused. (see Chapter 3).

At present, I can cope with the 'voices' during the daytime but it is at nights that there are difficulties. The 'voices' can wake you up at anytime during the night. There is a certain regularity. If the 'voices' do not wake me up in the middle of the night then they regularly wake me up at 4.30 in the morning. I spoke to Dr Carson about this persistence of schizophrenia but it is manageable. I get up and turn on the TV to distract me from the 'voices' and try to ignore the 'voices'. I learnt to *ignore* the 'voices' from John Nash in the film 'A Beautiful Mind'. I have other coping strategies which I have obtained through therapy including using cleaning as a means of coping with my illness. I am not free of the symptoms of schizophrenia but at least I am in the process of recovery. I hope that the therapy will lead to not having a major relapse leading to hospitalisation.

Comment

I have lived with schizophrenia for eighteen years. It is a strange period in one's life. From 1991 to 2001 I lived with the 'delusion' of Soviet mental communication. It is now in 2011 that I can say that I am surprised at my own mental health because I am a rationalist in my philosophical outlook apart from my interest in materialist dialectics. What I did during the period 1991 to 2001 was to rationalise my 'delusions' without telling anyone. From 2001 on I have taken a 'conscious' approach to my illness even though it did not prevent me from breaking down. From 2003 to 2011 I have lived with mild schizophrenia. I hear 'voices' but they are not severe and incessant. I can cope and have, through therapy, developed coping strategies to help me cope with the 'voices'.

*

In 2008, the problem with the 'voices' was that they talked about things that I did not understand and said some strange things to me, like talking to me about pumpkins. The 'voices' also talked to me about chess and gave me chess forms to try and solve. It is indeed strange how the brain works. The regularity of the 'voices' is seen in that they wake me up at four-thirty in the morning and start talking to me. I have to get out of bed and go to the front room and turn on the television to distract me from the 'voices'. I try to distract myself and ignore the 'voices,' because any involvement means not being able to recover. The next chapter is concerned with the journey of recovery and how I tried to make my life meaningful whilst living with schizophrenia.

References

Bellamy, J. (2000) Can you hear me thinking? *Psychiatric Rehabilitation Journal*, 24, 1, 73-75

Hegel, G. (1969) *Hegel's Science of Logic*. Translated by A. Miller. London: Allen and Unwin

3

My journey of recovery

Gordon McManus

In 2001, Gordon was diagnosed with paranoid schizophrenia. He decided to use writing and playing chess on his new computer, as two strategies to try and cope with his illness. In 2002, his father died. Four months after this, he had a relapse of his illness, and he was again Sectioned under the Mental Health Act. He found social acceptance at a club in Brixton, where he was respected for his chess and dominoes playing. When the club closed down, he offered to host the dominoes sessions in his own flat, where he also cooked for his friends. He started a book on Globalisation as a way of coping with his political 'voices,' which he eventually finished in 2006, four years after embarking on the project. It was also in 2006 that he was offered cognitive behaviour therapy sessions, at the Maudsley Hospital. This was his first introduction to the concept of recovery. The following year he started working with Jerome. Together they developed a model of Gordon's own recovery. In the chapter, Gordon also describes what he learned from influential figures in the wider recovery movement. Their work offered him inspiration. For Gordon, recovery can be described most succinctly as coping with your illness, whilst trying to have a meaningful life.

In 2001 when I came out of hospital I was diagnosed as paranoid schizophrenic by my consultant psychiatrist, Dr Jonathan Bindman. I did not know what to do. My carer, my sister, Laura, gave me two books on schizophrenia by health professionals. I read pages from them concerning case studies on those who were experiencing this disease. I resolved to 'rebuild' my life. I was given a computer by my youngest sister, Moira, and this technological device became a catalyst of change for me. I decided to use writing and playing the computer at chess in order to retrain my conceptual thinking, given that I had 'lost' this function during the 'schizophrenic phase' of my life. I decided on writing about politics in order to be 'rid' of political 'voices' and to understand why I became affected with schizophrenia because of politics. I had after nine years of suffering from schizophrenia a goal for 'rebuilding' my life

---

The first piece of writing that I completed using the computer, was on the Conservative Party leadership contest, which was won by Iain Duncan-Smith. During the period of schizophrenia, I could not fill out a form, let alone write on political matters. This was a new development for me. It was the first piece of writing I had done since 1992 when, at that time, I was writing about the implosion of Soviet socialism and the lessons to be learnt. I was also trying to overcome my 'anger' with the Left, especially the Communists in this country. I became more positive about my life. I gave a copy of my political writing to Dr. Bindman to show him that I was trying to 'rebuild' my life.

I also renewed my friendships with Karl and Eric during that year as I said to myself that schizophrenia should not stop me from being friends with them. I had allowed schizophrenia to dominate me too much. I had stopped being friends with Karl and Eric because of the 'voices.' This was another aspect of 'rebuilding' my life. In December of 2001, Karl came to me at The Studio which housed a social club run by a member of the Black British reggae group, Matumbi. The Studio was my social outlet during the 1990s and 2000. Karl asked for firstly a 'Marxist' explanation of Globalisation, and then qualified it by asking me about a 'Marxist-Leninist' explanation of Globalisation. I did not know the 'Marxist' explanation but I told him that for 'Marxism-Leninism,' Globalisation is Imperialism. It was simple because the highest stage of capitalism for Lenin is Imperialism and this the 'Marxist-Leninists' religiously follow. I decided to do research on 'Globalisation' from bourgeois theorists and communist parties. I used the computer and the Internet to research the matter. I 'surfed' the World Bank website, the International Monetary Fund, the Bank of England and the European Central Bank, to develop my understanding. I looked at the South African Communist Party website (SACP) and found an article where they declared that 'Globalisation is Imperialism'. I could now say to Karl that I was correct on the 'Marxist-Leninist' explanation, but was the 'Marxist-Leninist' explanation correct. The issue was 'What is Globalisation?' and was it Imperialism? This was the nucleus of my investigations.

I carried on my research in 2002. During this period I was still hearing 'voices' but they were not so severe.

In May 2002, my father passed away. I tried not to let it affect me. For the next three months I researched on Globalisation and I even took up driving lessons as I was 'voice-free'. In September the 'voices' came back heavily. I tried to cope with it. It was my sister, Laura, who detected that my behaviour was becoming irrational. I was not answering the phone because of the 'voices'. She got worried and entered the flat without my permission.

I threw her out. She spoke to my social worker, Charlene deVilliers. The social worker and my consultant psychiatrist Dr. Bindman, came to see me and advised me to enter hospital. I knew I was having a 'breakdown' but did not want to be hospitalised, so I refused. A few days later, my sister Laura, the social worker, the consultant psychiatrist and my GP, Dr. Bennett, came to see me and again advised me to go into hospital. I refused again. They then got the police and I was arrested and Sectioned under the Mental Health Act and was taken to the South-Western Hospital. I spent nearly three months in hospital. I came out of hospital in January 2003. I recount this episode because it 'arrested' the 'rebuilding' of my life. I have to say this: Was I correct in my approach or were they correct for putting me in hospital? I can now say that they were correct.

What does being hospitalised and sectioned mean? It means fighting to prove you are 'recovering' from your illness. It means convincing the Mental Health Tribunal that you are capable. Being sectioned means not being able to go out of the ward and being kept a close eye on by the nurses. It means that until the section order is lifted, you do not have liberty. It means a loss of goals in your life. It means loss of personality or identity. It means fighting for your goals and identity. It means the consultant psychiatrist and his/her team decide whether you have overcome your illness through medication. It means reliance on the 'medical model' of treatment. It means that leaving hospital becomes a goal at that stage of your life.

When you leave hospital you have to adjust to the pace of social reality as presented by your family and friends. Family and friends wonder whether you are able to achieve 'normality'. You yourself wonder whether you are capable of 'normality,' after two hospitalisations in three years. You have to cope with the stigma that exists within society over people who become mentally ill. It is not only your illness but social determinants that also affect your life. Well-being and being 'free of the symptoms' is a distant dream.

After two breakdowns in three years I did not know whether I could 'rebuild' my life. Was I always going to be plagued by schizophrenia for the rest of my life? I had to do something. I kept to my goals of writing and chess to rebuild my intellectual function. I was not 'free' of political 'voices' and there was still anger with the Left in Britain, both in terms of the political 'voices' and with the Left itself. For the next two years I had difficulty 'rebuilding' my life. I did research on Globalisation and used the World Bank website primarily as I 'thought' that it had the best discussion on the subject. I was having problems writing a thesis on Globalisation because I was coming to the conclusion that the 'Marxist-Leninist' argument that 'Globalisation is Imperialism,' was incorrect.

During these two years – from 2003 to 2004 – my social outlet was still The Studio. People who went there did not know that I suffered from schizophrenia and treated me as 'normal,' though somewhat eccentric. They respected me for my chess and my domino playing. Games like these two provided a distraction from the 'voices' and a focus on acting 'rationally'. I met Stanton Delgado (cousin of the late Jamaican reggae singer, Junior Delgado), Delroy Simpson (Simmo – cousin of the former Jamaican Prime Minister Portia Simpson Miller) and Keith Bent. We were the regular domino players and Stanton was responsible for organising events at The Studio. Keith and I formed one team, whilst Stanton and Zimmo formed the other team. When one team gave the other team '6-0', there was great rejoicing. I coined a term for such a beating, and that was 'Greetings'. The domino language for winning '6-0' was 'Greetings'. If I was having difficulties during the day at my flat with the 'voices,' it was to some extent negated by my 'sociality' at The Studio. Even Linton Kwesi Johnson and his son Eric would play dominoes. It made life bearable. In 2004, The Studio closed down. These friends encouraged me to write when I told them I was doing something on Globalisation. I was no longer purely 'engaged' with the 'voices.' I had outlets to 'rebuild' my life. Most of all I had **not** broken-down and been hospitalised.

In 2005, whilst I was still researching on Globalisation, I asked Stanton if he, Zimmo and Keith wanted to play dominoes at my place, because The Studio had closed down. I decided that this 'sociality' needed to occur at my place if I was to rebuild my life. They agreed. I provided the place and the food and they provided the 'sociality'. Stanton was asked to organise these events, which occurred fortnightly (see Chapter 5). Stanton proved himself a capable organiser which allowed me to 'rebuild' my life. The domino sessions gave me a 'routine' which brought a certain stability to my life. It did not make me isolated which schizophrenia usually leads to. We had discussions on Globalisation and Imperialism and I had to persuade them that Globalisation is **not** Imperialism. I was successful and this developed my writing.

Writing by 2005, had become important to me. It was not something that I fully committed to before in my life. It gave my life meaning. It gave me a sense of identity. It gave me a 'voice' – an expression of my views. It served as a means of 'distancing' me from the 'voices', from schizophrenia. There was still no book yet or even a manuscript. In late summer of 2005 the 'voices' became severe and the voice of Tony Blair, the Prime Minister at the time, became the most prominent. I resolved that I did not want a breakdown and hospitalisation. I gave myself the goal of writing a book and immersed myself in it in order to counter the 'voices' and to engage in my 'sociality'. This was a very important time. It was whether I would continue to 'rebuild' my life or live a life of schizophrenia. I had to fight this disease and thus I committed myself to writing a book on Globalisation.

For the next six months I developed a discipline which I had not had since the 1980s when I was teaching. Any time free of the 'voices' was given to writing apart from the 'dominoes sessions'. I was encouraged by my domino friends but they were getting impatient about the time taken. They, by the end of 2005, still did not know that I suffered from schizophrenia. I had told Keith in early 2002 that I suffered from 'depression,' but that was to explain why I was not working. Eric kept things to himself, as he knew. Eric, at that time, played a crucial role in my attempt to 'rebuild' my life. He showed concern when I was hospitalised in 2002. He provided an outlet that allowed me to 'rationalise' my life. We played chess despite my schizophrenia. I taught him chess again. I had stopped teaching him chess because of schizophrenia. The relationship with Eric improved my desire to return to 'normal life'. During this period my relationship with my family had improved a lot. My sister Laura did not want me to engage in political writing as she believed this would affect me, possibly making me 'more schizophrenic.' I was adamant I had to write because I had to be rid of 'political voices' and writing was the only means. Thus I carried on with my goal. I finished the 'book' around March-April 2006.

In the early part of 2006, Stanton, when he realised that not only had I written on Globalisation but also on Socialism and the State, said that I should set up a website publishing my writing on the Internet. I agreed with him and also said that I wanted to publish a monthly news sheet for my website. The aim was to distance myself from the 'political voices' by publishing my views on the Internet, instead of talking to the 'political voices' and forms. This act made feel 'normal' instead of being labelled 'schizophrenic'. The computer was enabling me to 'rebuild' my life while my domino friends were unaware that I suffered from schizophrenia.

During 2005, Dr McGowan became my consultant psychiatrist and he referred me for counselling therapy so that I could 'recover'. I learnt about this when I went to the Psychological Interventions for Psychosis (PICuP) Clinic at the Maudsley Hospital. It was the first time since my first hospitalisation in 1994 that I was given therapy. It had taken fourteen years. I started therapy in May 2006. It was the first time that I came across the concept of 'recovery'. Two years later, I asked Dr McGowan why he referred me for therapy and he said that medication was not working and that therapy might help. I am grateful to Dr McGowan for his care and consideration and thank him for it. It led to the phase of 'recovery' concerning my illness.

When the 'book' was finished I felt a certain cathartic relief. I was still not 'voice free'. I had learnt to cope with my illness. The therapy sessions were a 'God-send' (even though I am an atheist). They lasted for six months and every fortnight we would meet. I would talk about the 'voices' with my therapist, a counselling psychologist. She gave me coping strategies which I was not aware of before. She made me aware that there were people who coped with 'living with voices'. The importance of these sessions was that they prevented me from having a break-down and another hospitalisation. To 'talk' about my condition was very important to me. It gave me **hope** for 'recovery'. The only blight was when the Counsellor told me that 'schizophrenia is like cancer'. I first became distressed. It meant that there could not be 'full recovery,' which I was aiming for with these therapy sessions. I was walking to the bus stop from the Maudsley Hospital, when I looked up and saw my therapist's form and heard her voice. The distress had caused this to happen in the middle of the road. I thought I would be hospitalised but I managed to get home and get over this incident. I became depressed. This was the first time I felt 'depression'. I suffer from schizophrenia but not schizophrenia and depression at the same time. I spoke to my Community Psychiatric Nurse (CPN) Simon Gent. We talked about 'recovery'. He referred me for 'in-house' therapy with Dr Jerome Carson in late 2006. I would like to thank Simon Gent for his care.

In January 2007, I met Dr. Carson who conducted psychological tests on me to ascertain my condition. He came to the conclusion that I was schizophrenic and depressed. He decided to take my case up.

The first surprise for me was the discussion on 'recovery' with Dr Carson. In the first few months I came across Patricia Deegan (Deegan, 1996), Rachel Perkins (Perkins, 2006), Dr Peter Chadwick (Chadwick, 1993) and James Bellamy (Bellamy, 2000), amongst others. Patricia and James had suffered from schizophrenia from a young age and had written about their experiences. I was given two articles written by them. Dr Carson wanted me to read them. My first impression was that I was not like them. I did not suffer schizophrenia from a young age. I was in Dr Carson's, words 'late-onset,' which meant the possibility of 'full recovery'. However I decided to follow Dr Carson's advice. I read these articles on the bus going back home. I was surprised. When I got home I re-read them again. What impressed me was that they had confronted their illness. I had decided to 'rebuild' my life but I had not yet confronted my illness. James Bellamy's article made me aware of how other people have experienced schizophrenia and the social stigma that one is faced with (Bellamy, 2000). Deegan's article was based on her experiences and how she obtained a doctorate in psychology, because she did not like how she was treated (Deegan, 1996). She gives her definition of recovery which took me a long time to understand. It inspired me to write about my illness. I wrote a page and a half and showed it to Dr Carson as I tried to make sense of this new concept called 'recovery'. The next article I read and which was influential, was by Rachel Perkins, called 'you need hope to cope'. It was now that I consciously recognised that **coping** with my illness was the key to 'recovery' and that **hope** plays a very important role (Perkins, 2006). In 'recovery' hope and coping are two very important concepts. I felt like a psychology student rather than a person with schizophrenia'. The sessions with Dr Carson gave me a sense of 'self-purpose'. Dr Carson, through the concept of 'recovery' and the experiences of others, helped me confront and rationalise my illness. It is important to 'intellectualise' my illness as making it logical helps me to cope. It means restructuring my identity and my social role. It means 'coming to terms' with your experience and to make sure others benefit from it.

In October 2007, Dr. Carson said that I should do a public presentation on my 'Recovery'. I hesitated at first because I had not fully comprehended Deegan's approach and I did not feel ready yet but I eventually agreed with Dr. Carson as doing it would help my 'recovery'.

In November 2007, I confided to Stanton and the domino crew that I suffered from schizophrenia not simply depression. They accepted the fact. Keith wanted to know what it really meant. I told him that I heard voices and saw forms of people, including friends. He asked me whether I had heard 'voices' about him. I said 'Yes'. They, over the last two to three years had got to know me. They, the domino crew, had helped to 'rebuild' my human persona and I thanked them for it. I told them that I am not free of the symptoms but that the dominoes helped to 're-discover' myself. It is members of the Black (West Indian) Community through dominoes that have aided my 'recovery'. Stanton was surprised and he adopted an approach of 'psycho-analysing' me from his knowledge. I began to explain my condition to him. The domino sessions continued as they tried to treat me 'normally'. This gave me confidence and self-esteem.

In December 2007, things came together. I started to get to grips with Deegan. I began to comprehend her understanding of 'recovery' and was impressed. Dr Carson and I developed a model of recovery. The McManus/ Carson model of recovery begins with normal life. The next stage is the descent into mental illness which leads to a breakdown and hospitalisation. The third stage is the recovery period, which is coping with the illness and trying to develop a meaningful life. The fourth and final stage is concerned with resuming a normal life. It meant that I could understand the course of my life. This 'rationalisation' was very important. I felt better about doing a public presentation to the local Recovery Group, which Dr Carson had suggested.

In February 2008, I did the public presentation. It was a success. It was the first time as I have explained before that I have publicly talked or discussed my illness. There were over 20 people present, including my old social worker, Charlene deVilliers. True it was within the confines of the community mental health teambase, but I hoped that people would learn from my experiences. I was contributing to society again even though I was diagnosed with schizophrenia. It was, however, a stressful though fulfilling experience. I managed to 'keep my head' together during the presentation. For the next three days, I heard 'voices.' I did not know how I managed to answer questions and the effects of this took their toll. Stanton discussed the matter with me and it relieved the situation. It was only when I saw the film of the presentation that my sister's partner took, that I understood the magnitude of what I had done.

The year 2008 resulted in developing my understanding of 'recovery'. It meant looking at my achievements in life and not taking a negative view which is very important in recovering from schizophrenia. This year saw Dr Carson saying to me that he and I should write a book on my 'Recovery'. This chapter is a result of that discussion. This book is a result of that discussion.

I have to say that writing about my experiences concerning schizophrenia is part of my therapy in my 'recovery process'. I have, in writing the three chapters, had to fully confront my illness and rationalise my experiences. It is something that I need clarity for. Clarity is important to me as it lessens the stress of my illness.

Recovery: Is it feasible?

I would like to engage in the debate within the Mental Health Service concerning 'recovery' using my own experience.

First of all I have to mention that the method of treatment from my first hospitalisation in 1994 to 2005, was almost exclusively based on the 'medical model' which relies on medication as a means of recovery, as a cure. It was in 2006, that I first came across the concept of 'recovery,' when I attended therapy sessions at the PICuP Clinic. The treatment of my illness had changed. I was also receiving psychological treatment. Thus from

May 2006, my treatment consisted of both medication and psychological counselling. In my treatment both the medical model and the 'recovery' model complemented each other in the last two years.

My stage of 'recovery' has two phases to it. The first phase from 2001 to 2005 was based on the medical model of treatment. I call this phase the 'rebuilding' phase. I attempted to redevelop my intellectual functioning with the goal of returning to teaching, which was my occupation, in 2001. Moreover, for myself, schizophrenia practically destroyed my rational functioning. The sub-goals were writing and playing chess against the computer with the aim of playing competitive chess. Unfortunately, for me, I broke down in 2002 and was subsequently hospitalised. I came out of hospital in January 2003. For the next two years I had difficulty 'rebuilding' my life. In 2005, with the encouragement of the domino crew, I started writing again. I managed to finish the 'book' in March-April 2006. It was a goal that I had achieved in spite of my schizophrenia. I was playing chess but it was here that I was having difficulty. I could not get 'rid' of the chess 'voices' and forms. They were quite severe. It was only in 2008 that they have become 'mild'.

The second phase begins in May 2006 with my acquaintance with the concept of 'recovery'. However, it was only in January 2007 that I came to grips with it when I began therapy with Dr Carson. I began to understand the concept of 'recovery' in December 2007, just before my public presentation. It was under Dr Carson's 'tutelage' that I have an understanding of 'recovery'. He made me confront my illness and rationalise it, which is very important for my 'recovery'. The concept of 'recovery' became an intellectual tool for my recovery. What follows is my understanding.

'Recovery' is a goal. By definition, 'recovery' is an aim which the patient has to strive for. It means that the patient is determined to overcome his/her mental illness. Recovery is not a cure as Deegan points out. She states that:

> Recovery refers to the lived or real life experience of people as they accept and overcome the challenge of their disability... they experience themselves as recovering a new sense of self and of purpose within and beyond the limits of the disability. (Deegan, 1996)

Perkins substantiates this position:

> It is about recovering meaning, purpose and identity – about pursuing your interests and ambitions, and discovering new ones, in the presence of ongoing or recurring problems. (Perkins, 2006)

For myself, writing, chess and dominoes, were goals that I pursued. They gave me meaning, purpose and identity for my recovery whilst coping with my illness. It was, in relation to 'identity', having a 'new sense of self'. This was very important in my recovery and the dominoes session served this 'purpose' well. The development of the 'self' is very important in the 'recovery' process. You need 'hope to cope' and one of the great hopes is a 'new sense of self'. As Deegan points out:

> The goal of (recovery) is to become the unique, awesome, never to be repeated human being that we are called to be. (Deegan, 1996)

The 'sociality' of the domino sessions gave me a 'new sense of self'. It gave me a meaningful life with a sense of purpose. The domino sessions made us friends. I have developed a friendship with Stanton Delgado, which has surprised me. What schizophrenia had tried to destroy, was being overcome with these domino sessions. It was not only the domino sessions. It was also the food that I cooked. Stanton, Simmo, Keith and Karl were surprised at my culinary skills. They were aware of my writing and in this sense Simmo and Stanton gave me encouragement. These developments helped me 'distance' myself and 'ignore' the 'voices' as shown by Russell Crowe playing John Nash in the film, 'A Beautiful Mind'. These factors have helped to cope with my illness and to have a meaningful life. As Retta Andresen and her colleagues define 'recovery' as:

> The establishment of a fulfilling meaningful life and a positive sense of identity founded on hopefulness and self-determination. (Andresen et al, 2003)

Deegan, Perkins and Andresen and her colleagues, have all contributed towards a conscious understanding of 'recovery' in relation to my goals. This has made my life bearable because I am still not free of the symptoms of schizophrenia. The struggles of Deegan, Perkins and Dolly Sen (Sen, 2002; 2006), have inspired me to engage fully in the 'recovery' process. It is the only 'hope' in fully recovering from schizophrenia.

The concept of 'self determination' is very important in my opinion. It means being determined over the development of the 'self', of 'identity' and in the final analysis, the development of the 'personality' of the person who is affected by mental ill-health. This is Deegan's revolutionary contribution to the 'recovery' method of treatment. The development of the 'personality' of the mentally ill person must go hand in hand with 'sociality'. It means overcoming stigma about being mentally ill and this depends on friends and family. It means being open about your illness and not hiding it. For the years from 1994 to 2001, I hid my illness. I was diagnosed during this period as suffering with paranoid psychosis. It was only in 2001 that I told Dr Bindman that I lived with 'voices'. He diagnosed me with schizophrenia. I hid the fact that I suffered from schizophrenia from my domino friends for nearly three years from 2005 to 2007. It was only in late 2007 just before my public presentation that I revealed the truth about my condition. It was a relief to come out and be open about it. It helps one to 'recover'. I am lucky in that family and friends have stood by me despite my illness.

I raised the question about 'recovery' – is it feasible? It is not only feasible but a goal that a person with mental ill-health is striving for. It entails a new approach by mental health professionals be they psychiatrists, psychologists, community psychiatric nurses and social workers. They must be qualified with understanding the relationship between the medical model of treatment and the 'recovery' method of treatment. My 'improvement' came with being treated by both the medical model and the 'recovery' method. I have not had a breakdown leading to hospitalisation in the last few years.

The McManus/Carson model of recovery

I am someone who has a late onset condition. It means that I became mentally ill at a later age than most sufferers. It struck me in my early forties. Before that I had a normal life. My chosen occupation was being a teacher and teaching. I was also engaged in politics and played competitive chess whenever I had time from my political activity. I socialised by going to parties and functions. Politics was however primary in my life.

It was in 1991 that I first became mentally ill but I did not realise it at the time. I broke down in 1993, but this time my parents looked after me. I broke down again in 1994 and I was hospitalised. I was diagnosed first with paranoid psychosis and later with paranoid schizophrenia. This was the period of 'irrationality'. It means loss of personality and lack of care. It means lack of communication with people and being 'obsessed' with the 'voices'. It means being alienated from society and social life, including family. This is a difficult period where there is nothing of interest but the 'voices'. It meant a breakdown in my life leading to hospitalisation where the emphasis was on the 'medical model' of treatment.

In 2001 I decided to 'rebuild' my life. I, unknowingly, embarked on the stage of recovery. The stage of recovery has two phases to it: the first phase is

The McManus/Carson Model of Recovery

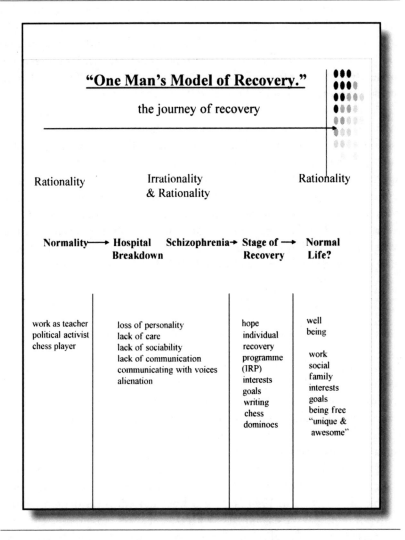

concerned with 'rebuilding' my life and was from 2001 to 2005. The mentally ill patient can regress. I had a breakdown and hospitalisation in 2002. The second phase, from 2006 to 2008, was concerned with 'recovery' and becoming conscious of coping with mental illness and having a meaningful life. I used my interests, for example, writing chess and dominoes, to have a meaningful life and at the same time having better relations with family and friends. It was my own **individual recovery plan.** I do not know how long this stage lasts. It may take years and it may take a short time. The goal during this stage is to cope with your illness and to have a meaningful life. It means you are not fully 'rational' but striving towards that goal.

The final stage is that of resuming 'normal life' or obtaining 'rationality'. It means being 'free of the symptoms' of your illness. It means well-being. It means being able to socialise and to work. This is material well-being. It means having good relations with your family and friends. It means having a social life. It means, as Deegan points out, being 'the unique, awesome, never to be repeated human being'. It means living a 'normal life' taking into account that the patient, in this case, myself, has experienced a period of mental ill health. It means the realisation of goals and interests that show the personality in its full expression. It means making up for the 'lost years' of your mental illness. This final stage is the goal of my 'recovery'.

This recovery model or my individual recovery plan (IRP) helps to objectify my mental illness. It enables me in 'trying times' to rationalise my condition. I live on a 'day-to-day' basis. I know that I can also regress, as occurred in the past. This model of recovery is, for me, a substantiation of the goals that I am striving for, no matter how long it takes.

At this juncture, I would like to express my gratitude to Dr Carson, my therapist. He helped by 'fleshing' the model out because I was not fully clear what I was doing or aiming for. He helped me 'rationalise' my condition and this gives meaning to my life. This enabled me to do the public presentation. It enabled me to articulate to people my condition and how I was trying to 'recover'.

The importance of this model of recovery is that there should be an individual recovery plan for each mentally ill patient. It enables the mentally ill to have goals to improve their life. It gives 'hope'. The 'hope' to fully recover is a goal worth striving for.

This model of recovery was inspired by Deegan's understanding of 'recovery'. She made me aware of having goals. Having goals helps you to cope better with your illness. Coping with your illness means having hope that you, yourself, will lead a meaningful life. This is what this model signifies for me.

Recovery, through this model, means for me coping with my illness, with the 'voices' whilst trying to have a meaningful life.

References

Andresen, R. Caputi, P. & Oades, L. (2003) The experience of recovery from schizophrenia: towards an empirically validated stage model. *Australian and New Zealand Journal of Psychiatry*, 37, 586-594

Bellamy, J. (2000) Can you hear me thinking? *Psychiatric Rehabilitation Journal*, 24, 1, 73-75

Chadwick, P. (1993) The stepladder to the impossible: A firsthand phenomenological account of a schizoaffective psychotic state. *Journal of Mental Health*, 2, 239-250

Deegan, P. (1996) Recovery as a journey of the heart. *Psychiatric Rehabilitation Journal*, 19, 3, 91-97

Perkins, R. (2006) You need hope to cope. In, Roberts, G. Davenport, S. Holloway, F. & Tattan, T. (Eds) *Enabling Recovery: The principles and practice of rehabilitation psychiatry*. London: Gaskell

Sen, D. (2002) *The World is Full of Laughter*. Brentwood: Chipmunka Press

Sen, D. (2006) *Am I still Laughing?* Brentwood: Chipmunka Press

4
Working with Gordon:
Perspectives from mental health
professionals

Charlene DeVilliers, Jonathan Bindman, Daisy Masona, Claudette Miller as told to Sophie Davies

Charlene, Gordon's social worker and care co-ordinator at the start of the last decade, talks about the work needed to re-establish him in the community, after his section admission. Charlene helped get Gordon's benefits restarted and his flat redecorated. Having seen Gordon at his most unwell, it was a pleasant surprise for her when she heard him talk about his model of recovery in his first public presentation some years later. Dr Jonathan Bindman takes up the theme of how people change dramatically, as was the case with Gordon, when they are psychotic. He points out that the more ill a patient is, the more likely they are to have greater contact with the psychiatrist. As a patient recovers, they are likely to see less of their psychiatrist. Both Charlene and Jonathan worked with Gordon when he was at his most unwell. Claudette saw Gordon move slowly into his recovery journey and noticed changes in him over a period of years. She draws our attention to Gordon's humility and gentleness and his ability to communicate with people at different levels. Finally, Daisy has worked with Gordon most recently, when he has been relatively well. She has been impressed with his optimism and commitment to his recovery. She sees a wider message in this improvement as she comments, 'Gordon and others are breaking free of the gravitational pull of this illness in their quest for freedom.'

Charlene DeVilliers: The social worker's story

Gordon only came to the attention of the services of 380 Streatham High Road in 2001, even though he had been ill for a long time. It was obvious by the time he became re-involved with services he was really quite ill. It was a shame that he hadn't been picked up by services before that point. However, he may not have sought out our help because his family had been looking after him. Also he may have been reluctant to get involved with services on a personal level.

The admission was difficult. The police picked up Gordon on the street carrying a knife, which was obviously quite worrying. Fortunately though, he was open to being involved with services. That's when I became involved in Gordon's care as his social worker and care coordinator.

We took a task-centred approach to Gordon's treatment at first, because it seemed that he had been neglecting things he needed to do for quite a while. This was because he'd been deteriorating and finding it hard to undertake day-to-day jobs. I helped him to maximise his benefits for instance, which he needed help doing.   We also sorted out Gordon's flat, which needed redecorating. We applied for four grants and got an organization to come in and do the redecorating work for him. The flat looked really good afterwards and Gordon was really proud of how smart it looked. It's always nice to have a good environment, as it can make you feel better about yourself, and this was certainly the case for Gordon. He does spend a fair amount of time in his flat too – he likes to do research on his computer. Gordon was living on his own at this time, though his sister Laura came to visit a lot.

Things were going okay at this point and Gordon was starting to admit to his friends that he suffered from schizophrenia. This was good news because it signified that he was being open about his illness. He was working towards recovery but was still preoccupied with his globalisation interests and still doing lots of researching of Marxist and Leninist ideas. Those interests remained a large part of my regular discussions with him, but of course I didn't want to discourage these pursuits entirely, because they were part of who Gordon was.

He was still playing a lot of dominoes with friends too, so I encouraged him to carry on doing that, as social interaction was a positive. A lot of work was about trying to give Gordon more structure and a daily routine. That was quite hard for him because he wanted to be heavily involved in his research interests still. However it was necessary for us to monitor this to make sure that he was attending to his daily tasks and visiting his family. He said that he was taking his medication at this point. However it's always hard to know whether someone is or not - even when people say they are, this is sometimes not the case.

Gordon's father died in 2002, and the build-up to his father dying was a big thing. He had been ill for a long time and Gordon was thinking a lot about this and whether he had let his father down. There were lots of feelings of remorse and guilt and he started to question if he had achieved all his goals in life. This was a really significant time for Gordon and I wonder in retrospect whether we should have organized bereavement counselling or similar for him to work through that period. Then, a while after his father died, Gordon said that he was completely free of 'voices.' But we had to question that. He was both quite elated and in denial about his father's passing away. Later in 2002 Gordon broke down and had a severe relapse. I remember that episode very well. He was having visual and auditory hallucinations all at once. It is very unusual to experience both at the same time. It showed how ill Gordon had become. He stopped going out, eating or attending to his care. He also stopped coming to see me and Dr Bindman. I remember I went to see him and told him that he needed to go and see Dr Bindman for review, but he didn't go to that either. Following this, we paid a visit to Gordon and felt that he hadn't improved. We decided at that point that hospital was the only option.

To get Gordon into hospital, we needed to section him. It was quite a tricky sectioning, because Gordon was very against the idea of being admitted. Sectioning someone is always hard because you need to have the police present at assessment, as well as find a bed in a hospital for someone and make sure that an ambulance is ready and so on. It was also difficult because he was my patient and I was having to drag him into hospital against his will. Laura was present too and she was obviously very, very upset. Gordon, for his part, was angry. He simply didn't want to be there. He kept on demanding to know why we had taken him there and saying that he didn't want to be in hospital. All in all, he was very hostile, which is completely the opposite of his normal demeanour. Gordon is usually a very calm, gentle and intellectual sort of man...but he turned so angry. I went onto his ward with Laura one time and he tried to attack his own sister. It was a very sad scenario. It was as though he wanted somebody to blame for being forced to be there. If I remember correctly, he also tried to assault one of the ward doctors. He was very aggressive with the nurses too and would just refuse to communicate with them. He didn't want to be involved in any group programmes. Rather, he simply wanted to lie in bed. When the nurses went up to him, he'd shout at them, which was not like Gordon at all.

It took a while for the medication to kick in but once it did – and it helped that he was given injections, rather than needing to take tablets himself – he started to improve really quickly. Gordon is very treatment responsive. Once he gets the treatment he requires he reacts very well. He was discharged home on a depot and I stopped seeing him. For around the next five years he was very well and much more stable than before. In 2007 he began to see Dr Jerome Carson, taking part in the recovery programme, and got even better. Participation in the recovery programme was a great idea for improving Gordon's social inclusion, and he says himself that he thinks it has had a positive effect on him, which is great.

Compared to other people diagnosed with schizophrenia Gordon's recovery has been very successful. He lives independently in his own flat, has some structure, has been very actively involved in the recovery programme and has some form of social life. Sadly he doesn't consider himself that he has 100% recovered yet, and as it was fairly late onset schizophrenia he can remember a time when he was completely well, and was living normally, lecturing and travelling and so on. That's very sad, yet his recovery really has been excellent compared to other sufferers.

In February 2008, I saw Gordon again at the local Recovery Group, an event organized as part of the Centre's recovery programme. Service users got to tell their own stories, which was really good because as a mental health practitioner you hardly ever get the chance to listen to the patients themselves telling their stories. It was a very, very interesting experience. Gordon spoke eloquently about his time in hospital, describing how difficult the period leading up to the sectioning was for him. It became clear how deeply affected he had been by his father's death. I remember him saying that he hadn't really foreseen how major an impact it would have on him. He also did admit to me that he hadn't been taking his medication as meticulously as he could have been during that period.

It was good hearing Gordon talk about his fears and ambitions. He still didn't feel his recovery journey was over and was keen on writing, reading, improving his knowledge and understanding and being further involved in the recovery programme. It was also really satisfying to see his confidence in talking in front of a room full of strangers. The room was packed. He did so well.

Gordon is a really amazing person. As a social worker, you meet hundreds of patients and hundreds of professionals, but when you meet Gordon you realise what an incredible journey he's been on and how far he has come. You can't help noticing how well he's done. Indeed, Gordon's a real role model and inspiration and it was fantastic to see him give his talk that day. It was also comforting to see his relationship with Jerome. They were relating to each other very much as equals – it wasn't a top down doctor-patient relationship.

Overall it was tough being both Gordon's care coordinator and his social worker because it meant I had to juggle those two roles in my head the whole time. You are always trying to think of alternatives to admitting somebody to hospital – by trying to improve their daily routine, undertaking relapse prevention work, trying to find out what the triggers of their illness are, to name but a few examples – but, at the end of the day, if someone becomes very ill you have to conclude that what they actually need more than anything is a hospital admission. That's no simple thing. There's all the paperwork, all the applications. We had to go to the court for a warrant as Gordon refused to open the door to us. We had to force our way in with the police, then once he was in hospital we had to explain his situation to the ward staff and read Gordon his rights and so on. It's a huge responsibility. There are so many things to juggle and ultimately, as the social worker, it's all on your head. Also, as care coordinator you are close to the person, so that makes it even harder. Now things have changed. Since the last Mental Health Act other people, like psychologists and nurses, can also take responsibility for sectioning someone, which is a welcome relief for social workers in such a complex area of mental health work.

Dr Jonathan Bindman: The psychiatrist's story

It was 2002, and we were on a freezing cold walkway. We finally managed to get into the flat. Gordon did not make eye contact and was furious. This was completely different to how he was before, which was distressing. I must have done hundreds of sectioning visits before, but you never get over the feeling of someone you thought you get on with just raging at you, not engaging and not acknowledging in any way that you had a relationship with them previously. Logically you think, well of course...they're psychotic. Why should they have a perception of reality that is the same as ours? Why should they be warm and friendly? And yet, so often when you have a relationship with somebody – and they have terrible 'voices' or delusions or hallucinations or whatever it may be – the human engagement normally survives. It's a shock when it's completely gone and that person becomes utterly hostile.

As a consultant you're not always well-placed in terms of understanding recovery because you mostly see people who are at 'crisis' point -- or those who cause the greatest concern to the team -- so you spend by far the most time with people who are doing badly. You also have the longest relationships with those who are doing particularly badly, going through repeated admission cycles, or who are generally very distressed. Whereas if someone starts to settle down and do better you see less of them. For someone like Gordon, the better he was, the less the consultant had to do with him. As a result, a lot of psychiatrists end up being slightly nihilistic or negative in their attitude towards recovery because they feel that schizophrenia means that you tend to relapse, that things tend to go badly.

There are some long-term studies showing that about one third of people who have a psychotic episode never have another, and another third recover quite well for long periods of time but maybe have short relapses. There's a final third who do chronically badly. If you look at the way consultant psychiatrists divide their time, they spend no time at all with those that have only one episode. They tend to see those that have relapses quite a bit when they are in crisis, particularly if they work in hospitals, but see them much less when they are at their best. If they are community based, they often have long term relationships with those who are chronically disabled. The picture you get is therefore completely skewed and that in turn tends to make you fear the worst.

There is an interesting debate going on in the critical psychiatry group about why we use such high doses of medication when the evidence to substantiate its efficacy is not terribly strong. High doses of medication are used because if you see a skewed group of people who relapse badly and often, you will naturally feel that medication is extremely important and that it is important for patients to stay on it, and you'll tend to apply that thinking to people who do not necessarily need such high doses of medication. There is the need for psychiatrists to be given more hope and positive messages which they can pass onto patients rather than passing on nihilistic messages.

Psychiatrists can have a terribly crude approach to insight. It is often assumed that if people are basically resisting treatment then they lack insight, whereas in fact the reasons people resist treatment may come from a whole range of different perspectives. Gordon, for instance, identifies strongly as a black man living in Brixton and is critical of institutions of power. From that perspective, the scenario in which a white middle class doctor comes, with the police, to the door of somebody who sees himself as a black man living in Brixton -- and we break the doors down and drag him off to a psychiatric institution-- has a whole lot of resonances quite separate from the question of mental illness. When it comes to insight therefore you might have a group of people who don't like being treated by mental health authorities because they see it as disempowering and oppressive rather than about being helped for psychotic symptoms.

One aspect of insight is sometimes said to be the ability to re-label symptoms. For instance if you hear a 'voice,' to say that's not the devil, that's a 'voice,' a psychotic 'voice,' that's only my illness that's talking to me, it isn't real. I think probably Gordon did not maintain that insight at all times because at the end of 2002 his 'voices' emerged and instead of saying to somebody 'the voice has returned, what can I do about it?' he became incredibly withdrawn and isolated. Only after a couple of weeks in hospital and medication was he able to admit that he had that 'voice,' didn't like it, and was doing something to get rid of it. Another aspect of insight is acknowledging, not just the symptoms of psychosis, but the illness itself. I think that Gordon did have a high degree of insight into that aspect of his problem. This is why he's become such an important figure in local recovery groups. Then comes the question of whether one takes prescribed medication for the problem.

The reason for breaking down insight into these three areas: re-labelling symptoms, accepting the problem and taking medication, is because it's possible to think and feel about those three areas very independently. You could acknowledge, for example, that you are hearing 'voices' but not consider it a problem and so not take medication. Or you might accept that you do have an illness, but not take medication because the side effects are unacceptable to you.

It is important to consider a patient's insight using these criteria. Gordon, even when he wasn't very well at all, could be engaged to some extent on whether he had a problem. He didn't like living in squalor and recognized that he had an illness. However, his insight seemed to vary a fair amount on the question of labelling his symptoms, that's to say, labelling the 'voices' he heard as a symptom of psychosis. In terms of medication, he seemed to have a fairly positive attitude towards it in 2001 but in 2002 something changed. It would be interesting to find out why he stopped taking medication.

It is always worth finding out if there are other reasons why people don't take medication. Sometimes they just forget, which is natural. But it is often written off as a lack of insight when, in reality, a lot of people stop taking medication quite simply because it means they gain weight or feel lethargic; men may not be able to get an erection or women feel effects on their libido or menstrual cycle. For these reasons, people may stop wanting to take medication but they may not tell the doctor why. Insight is often treated quite crudely yet it has quite a lot of depth. Gordon, fortunately, had quite a lot of insight at many levels, even when he was hostile, so you could work with him on how to improve things.

Claudette Miller: The team leader's story

I've known Gordon going back as far as 2003 as a member of the care coordination team and then as team leader. As a member of the team, I attended to him by administering depot medication. My main recollection of Gordon at that time was that he was very anxious about depot injections and required lots of reassurance. He also showed this sort of timidity and fear towards having an injection. He'd been on depot for a long while. I suppose injections can be quite unpleasant. It's the fear of having a needle that he had more than anything else. There were alternatives to the depot but in terms of consistency and maintenance, the injection was the best option. Once you've had the injection you can forget about medication for the next two or three weeks and you know it's going to consistently be in your system.

Despite needing lots of reassurance Gordon talked quite a bit, so in that sense the whole process was made quite a bit easier. I found him to be very warm and eloquent and a very knowledgeable man. His background was as a lecturer but, despite that, he was able to come down to a level where you felt a connection with him. The fear was the needle, which was quite long. For anyone that knows Gordon he's not a very big or meaty man, he's fairly slight. Once you had reassured him, he was fine and would take the medication because he also saw the benefits in terms of maintaining his health, and also allowing him the freedom not to have to take tablets every day. He needed greater reassurance in the injection being given than in the actual benefits of it.

Gordon was always humble, gentle when I met him. What really struck me was that he was really quite reserved in terms of his knowledge and experiences. He could talk at any level and I think because he was quite an intellectual person in terms of his background he wasn't aggressive in any way. Although he had this fear when you were administering an injection, you didn't feel at all unsafe when you were with him. You could see potential for him getting a lot better and moving through the system. You could also see that he understood his illness and that he got why he needed to take medication; not just the physical medication, but also involvement in other activities like the talking therapy. At times I remember he was a bit reluctant to get involved in structured daytime activities around that time but it was something you could change. Gordon was never rigid. I found that he was always very amiable and supportive in terms of what we were trying to do. I don't recall having any discussions with Gordon in terms of recovery at that stage. Our emphasis was not on recovery as such; we were providing care coordination/case management for service users. This meant looking at how to support and encourage Gordon to improve his quality of life, help him to get involved in more meaningful activities, comply with his treatment and expand his social life by looking at what was out them to help him, for instance day care centres.

Gordon's confidence has really improved; he's able to stand up now in front of people and speak. He has taken a very communicative role in his recovery with Jerome. You can see how he has grown from being someone who was sat, anxious to take his medication, to being someone who is able to talk about where he is at in his own recovery.

Through work in the recovery programme, he's got a lot of his self-esteem back and you can see that he's looking to the future. That is also reflected in his writing. It is evident that he now enjoys sharing his own life experiences in order to enable others to start to look at their own recovery. You can still lead a fairly normal life, that's to say – a life that is normal to you – and be in recovery. His collaboration with Jerome is one of the best things that has happened to Gordon because it's given him a life back, it's given him a purpose, a meaning, direction, as well as a platform to tell his own story etc, not just in this part of the Trust but in other areas too. He's really achieved a lot, from the day he was sectioned, to today. He is one of our success stories because he has not actually been in the red zone. The red zone is for clients we are really concerned about and who we think might need weekly, or even daily, discussions. In the amber zone, service users tend to be fairly stable though they typically still need quite a lot of input. The green zone is for users who are very well and who we would perhaps consider moving out of the service. With a total caseload of over 300, there are around 30-40 in the green zone. Gordon is currently in that zone.

In our role as care coordinators, we are in an excellent position to maintain service users' level of wellness and also point them in the direction of social inclusion. The latter is a very important part of our role. Normalization is also a crucial part of what we do. We look at individuals in terms of where they perceive they are at in their own recovery even before we start looking at a formal recovery model. Personal recovery is where they see they are at, instead of how we perceive it. As such we can't group everyone into the same category. With Gordon, you could see that in terms of intellect he was quite preserved i.e. he knew that if he didn't continue with the treatment programme the likelihood was that he would relapse, and that if he relapsed it was likely that his liberty might be taken away. It is not intended to be a threat; rather it's about giving someone information so that they are aware of the importance of complying with treatment. It's also a question of encouraging someone to be involved with social activities, to help them maintain some element of independence as well as inclusion in the community. That is another way of helping them to come out of the illness that they have. Powers of persuasion are therefore very important to the role of care coordinator. We want them to see that they are not alone in moving through the system, and to make them aware of all the choices that they have.

One of the drawbacks of our role is the limited time we have in providing the support that we feel someone like Gordon would benefit from. Another drawback is that, because care coordinators have a very high caseload, the time they have to look into what resources are available is very limited. In addition, historically it has been considered that people with schizophrenia can't engage in talking therapy. However research has shown that they can, and even if you provide just ten minutes, it's beneficial. I think we need to look more at that option for service users. With Gordon, although we were not formally giving therapy, when he talked to me or another care coordinator during the administering of the depot that was a kind of talking therapy. But it's about the relationship you build with service users and the support you give them in terms of helping them to better understand their symptoms, treatment and other services with which they can engage. For Gordon, the work with Jerome functions in the same way, but is more formal. What I hear a lot of service users saying, even if they are not saying it verbally, is simply, 'listen to me.' For a lot of service users, it's not that they don't want to take the medication, but rather, the physical effect it's having on them makes them not want to take it. It affects people in different ways. So it's about listening to service users and trying to make it comfortable for each of them. A lot might not be compliant due to the nasty side effects more than anything else, as well as the stigma attached to being on medication. It's a question of managing that.

Daisy Masona: The mental health nurses's story

I felt privileged when I was approached by Dr Carson to contribute to Gordon's book. Central to the story of Gordon, who is rightfully considered to be a 'recovery hero', is his optimism and resilience in pursuing his own recovery from a serious mental illness. Gordon wholeheartedly embraced the concepts of the recovery model and, with the formidable support of Dr Carson and the unwavering compliance of his medication regime, managed to transcend the limitations imposed by his illness. According to Professor Bill Anthony (1993), 'Recovery is a deeply personal unique process of changing one's attitude…involves the developing of new meaning and purpose in one's life.' This indeed is the story of Gordon who coined his own definition of recovery as 'coping with your symptoms and trying to have a meaningful life.' Gordon has resiliently lived up to this assertion.

My direct contact with Gordon was initiated when I joined the Recovery and Support team as the medication and depot clinic practitioner. Gordon was already functioning well in the community and attending the clinic fortnightly. In my capacity as Gordon's care coordinator it was within my remit to administer Gordon's two weekly depot injections, conduct ongoing mental state and risk assessments; monitor side effects of his medication and assess ongoing needs whereby appropriate action would be taken, if needed.

My predecessor had informed me about the service users who regularly attended the clinic, highlighting their current needs and diagnoses. My first impressions of Gordon were formed when I read through his medical records prior to meeting him. I was fascinated by the achievements of this academic, who had reached considerable heights in the political arena and had authored books after being diagnosed with a psychotic illness. Hence I was looking forward to meeting him with great anticipation. A good rapport was soon established between Gordon and myself.

One of the most important aspects of managing psychosis is to ensure compliance with medication, in order to prevent relapse in mental state. Throughout my work with Gordon, he diligently attended all his appointments. In fact he would arrive early and sit for an hour waiting for the depot to be delivered and administered. This was a brave action for someone who had a fear of injections. Gordon insightfully stated that he continued with his medication because it made him mentally stable. He also believed that if he was not compliant the professionals responsible for his care might believe that he was relapsing and he would find himself back in hospital. I believe Gordon was put on depot medication because of non-compliance issues in the past. I can confidently say that this is no longer an issue with Gordon, who participated in the making of Michelle McNary's Recovery Film (see www.slam.nhs.uk/patients/recovery.apsx) and in the writing of a book, among other life-fulfilling activities. I was glad to learn that Gordon is now on the tablet form of his medication, so will maintain his recovery without the pain of injections.

Gordon says that he is not free from the symptoms of schizophrenia but is in the process of recovery. He acknowledges that this is a personal journey which requires one's own commitment as well as the unflagging support of those involved in one's recovery. Gordon is determined to cope with his symptoms and to live a meaningful life. I ceased being Gordon's care coordinator when I moved from the Recovery and Support Team to the Assessment and Brief Treatment Team. However, I often catch a glimpse of Gordon and exchange a smile or a greeting when he attends for appointments. I recently had the pleasure of engaging in a conversation with Gordon several months after I stopped working with him. Gordon reiterated to me his desire to never get sectioned again.

Gordon's optimism and commitment to his recovery remains exemplary. He has fully embraced the new and innovative ways in which mental health problems are now managed, which defy the traditional gloomy prognosis of schizophrenia. Gordon singles out his therapy with Dr Carson as being instrumental to his continued recovery. Thanks to his model of recovery, he now has a structured life and is engaged in meaningful life-enhancing activities. Family ties are intact and he is supportive towards his widowed mother whom he phones daily.

The advent of atypical antipsychotic medication, with fewer side effects and more potency, has enhanced compliance with medication in service users. I used to administer one of these newer medications to Gordon. He did not experience any negative side effects. In the past one used to see patients gravitate towards increased morbidity and dysfunction under the debilitating side effects of typical antipsychotics, with little or no hope of recovery. It is true to say that the profession is experiencing a sense of professional fulfilment in witnessing service users, who are learning to cope with their symptoms and maximizing their strengths. Recovery stories are with us.

During our interactions I discovered that Gordon was a resourceful, insightful man who was able to draw from his inner strength and utilise professional interventions and his intellectual capabilities to resist the invading symptoms of a severe mental illness. It is important to note that Gordon applied the concepts of the recovery model well before it was ever introduced to him by Dr Carson in 2007. Gordon lucidly told me about when he was first diagnosed as schizophrenic in 1994. This was followed by several breakdowns and four hospitalisations until 2003. Thankfully this was his last hospitalisation. A vibrant thread of hope now runs through the prognosis of schizophrenia through the concerted efforts of health professionals and new trends of management as informed by research. Gone are the days when one would be left floundering for a response when a patient or a concerned carer asked about the prognosis of a major mental illness, because neither hope nor recovery fitted into the equation.

Gordon's delusional beliefs were linked to his political activities and yet he could not distinguish this aspect of his illness in the past. Gordon was initially overwhelmed by political voices and tried to get rid of them by putting them down on paper. Indeed, writing had a calming effect on him. Hence Gordon actively resisted drifting from a coherent social life by writing and organising a group of friends to meet weekly for a game of dominoes over curry. He embarked on extensive research into globalisation and wrote his book, which is not yet published. His family was very supportive and made it possible for Gordon to function fairly well without professional help long after he became unwell.

Although a diagnosis of schizophrenia is initially devastating, derailing and disruptive to one's future, we now have ample evidence of positivity, hope and recovery in many. Gordon and others are breaking free from the gravitational pull of this illness in their quest for freedom. I firmly believe that more and more service users will soon be able to function well in society with concerted high-level support from professionals.

Reference

Anthony, W. (1993) Recovery from mental illness: guiding vision of mental health service systems in the 1990s. *Psychosocial Rehabilitation Journal*, 16, 4, 11-23.

5
Knowing Gordon: Perspectives from family and friends

Eric Ayalande Johnson, Karl Miller, Stanton Delgado, Keith Bent, Gloria Giraud and Sophie Davies

This chapter starts with an interview conducted in Gordon's flat on a hot summer's evening. Karl, Stanton and Keith make up the dominoes crew, who meet every two weeks at Gordon's. He cooks them a meal and they play dominoes and chat all evening. Karl was at university with Gordon. He met Keith and Stanton through a social club called The Studio. After The Studio closed, they decided to carry on meeting and playing their dominoes. The warmth of their friendship and respect for Gordon shone though the interview, and it felt like a real privilege just to be there. Eric Ayalande Johnson, was the only friend that had contact with Gordon in periods when he was acutely ill, though he tells us in his account, that Gordon would often curse and swear at him during these times and refuse contact. Eric talks of the role that Gordon has played in his own life as a mentor and a friend, who taught him chess, helped with his poetry and explained Marxist principles. The final contribution is from Gordon's sister, Gloria Giraud. Gloria talks of the shock in the family when Gordon was first diagnosed with schizophrenia. She too stresses his personality characteristics of humility, gentleness, patience, kindness and understanding, and feels that now, 'there is a bright light at the end of that very long tunnel.'

Karl Miller, Stanton Delgado, Keith Bent, Gordon, Sophie and Jerome in conversation

... the dominoes crew interviewed in Gordon's flat.

Jerome: Tell us about when you first knew Gordon.

Keith: I first met Gordon in the late 1980s/early 1990s, at a little studio we used to go to in Brixton. I didn't really know Gordon personally but I knew him at that time to be one of the characters in the area. I knew him as a friend of Linton Kwesi Johnson, but also as one of the characters that used to frequent the place. He was one of those people who only spoke if he had something to say. I wasn't that close to him or a very good friend but we always said hello and asked how each other we're doing, and we shared the same space.

Then I started to notice after a while that Gordon removed himself from us in the same environment and I didn't quite know why. He would come in, buy himself a drink and have no communication with anyone, and I thought that was really strange. Even though I didn't know him very well I'd always say hello and good night. Then because I was such a bad chess player he'd show me how to play – but I still didn't know him that well at that time. Sometimes you'd get people in The Studio who didn't want to say anything, they'd just be there for the atmosphere, and I thought that maybe that was just the mood that Gordon was in.

Over the chess sessions we got to know each other a lot more and then when The Studio closed he started asking me to his flat to play and then we started speaking more in-depth about what he'd been going through in the last few years, things about his history, especially his involvement in the movement. It gave me a better understanding of Communism, of Marxism, of all those things that he was educated in for many years and I think he taught me a lot in terms of how I see the political world.

I've also grasped a fuller understanding of people who have experienced the same sorts of problems as Gordon. Previously I might have been one of those people who was indifferent towards a reclusive stranger. Gordon has changed me in that way, in the way that I view those people. You just don't know what is in people's minds, what's causing them to be like they are. And Gordon and I have a lot in common. I don't see Gordon as having an illness. I know he's on a recovery programme but I don't come round here thinking that I'm going to see a friend of mine who is sick.

Jerome: Have you ever met anyone before who's had this illness?

Keith: No...well I say no, but I've been around people who have suffered from schizophrenia and depression but I've never really been involved with them. I'm sure there are lots of people out there who have some of the symptoms but who haven't been declared 'sick' yet. You just handle people the way you find them. If Gordon was being a bit of an idiot I'd treat him a slightly different way, but he's a guy I've come to know and understand.

Karl: He's very strong-willed and opinionated. It really was a surprise to me when I heard about Gordon's illness. I mean I thought he had depression, but not schizophrenia. The thing is a lot of people involved in left-wing politics do tend to have mental illness problems. We used to know each other from way back at Essex University, we used to organise things together.

Jerome: So did you stay in touch after the Essex years?

Karl: Yes we did. We shared a flat together at one time. And he went and got all these books and he started playing chess and he got really good. I always take my hat off to him for that. I didn't know about a lot of the political stuff he was up to around that time, but I was glad to hear about it, especially the involvement in the anti-apartheid movement. I didn't agree so much with his communism. We've always been in touch. I think of all the university people, it's Gordon I've stayed in touch with the most.

Jerome: Karl, given that you knew Gordon for 20 years before he became ill how did you make sense of what was happening to him?

Karl: You know on the Left there's a fear – a sixth sense – that the State is going to get you. As you know the State kills more people around the world than anything else...so I guess I would put it down to that. But also with Gordon it was the difference between the reality and what he thought. Gordon is a very strong-willed person, with very strong ideas that he just won't let drop, and he was surrounded by people who would just let him have those ideas.

Keith: What I think is that throughout all the problems Gordon lost confidence in his own spirituality and he lost confidence in himself. In the last five years, Gordon has come back – not all the mishmash of what Gordon was supposedly fighting for – but Gordon himself has come back.

Karl: I think Gordon took too much on too. I think poverty probably had something to do with it too. I'm a great believer in poverty creating mental illness.

Sophie: Did you know each other continuously over all those years? Was there a gap at all?

Stanton: There wasn't a gap. I first met Gordon in 1997/ 98. My Mum had opened a sweet shop local to The Studio. A friend of mine had introduced me to The Studio, and I fell in love with it. The first time I stepped in there, it was like I'd stepped off earth. No one could find you, you were around people you wanted to be around. It was just a great place to be for socializing and the conversation in there was unreal – with all these different people from different walks of life. You could have great discussions.

When I first met Gordon I used to sit at the bar and have a chat with everyone. It was at the time when Gordon used to come in, order his drink and sit by himself. He'd sometimes talk to himself or he'd get quite angry with the TV or someone in the place. He'd vent his anger to himself in the corner, and I'd watch from afar. I wouldn't judge though. I didn't understand enough to be able to judge or have an opinion on what I'd seen. I think it was the middle of 1998 when I took more of an interest in the dominoes. The guys used to come and play and we'd pitch up and have a game. At that time Gordon was playing a lot more chess. You could see the change in his behaviour because he'd gone from sitting on his own doing nothing, having a drink and going home, to coming in and engaging. Then Gordon brought himself to the dominoes table where many epic battles were fought, won and lost. It was a great time.

Sophie: You didn't know at this stage that he was suffering from schizophrenia?

Stanton: No, no, I had my suspicions but nothing had been confirmed to me from Gordon or from anyone else who came to the place. I know loads of people who are suffering from depression and I don't consider them ill. I just think they're going through a bad time and you support them and you think they'll get better. I suppose that was my form of ignorance too because I didn't really understand what they were going through. I didn't realise the severity and the levels of depression until I became more intimate with Gordon and even then that didn't really happen until The Studio closed, which we were just sort of distraught about. All we could really think about was 'where are we going to play dominoes?' So we organized continuing the dominoes outside of the studio and starting something new. To be honest I didn't think it would take off. I just thought we'd get a couple of games in then it would fizzle out. The first session was held at my flat and it was a good night. I think it was the first time that Gordon had gone out and been somewhere that wasn't The Studio but he felt comfortable enough to come to my place and play dominoes. However we discovered that it wasn't the right venue and so that's when Gordon became the host. We've been playing constantly for five or six years now, every other Thursday.

Keith: It's the only thing I know I'm doing every other week! My friends, my family, know I play dominoes every other Thursday night. Any other night they don't know where I am or what I'm doing. It's our social event. Gordon speaks about how much it has helped him and how much we support him, but of course it gives us a night out too and the fact that we can sit around and chat seriously, chat rubbish if we want to, have a laugh and a joke, you know...it takes some of the edge off life, if you like. It's a great atmosphere to be in. Now, that might help Gordon, but it helps me too. Gordon's come back into our little reality by being able to take some things with a pinch of salt and not being able to find an answer for everything...you just can't always find an answer for everything.

Karl: Also in terms of Gordon's social circle, London is, like all the cities, a very lonely place.

Keith: Also Gordon grew up in the black community and black people can be very unsympathetic towards people who have a problem like that, because either they've got their own problems or they see it as a degrading sort of thing. There was another guy who used to just come in the studio and stare at people. I think he was on medication of some kind but no one tried to get around what his problem was or anything. People just used to think he was weird.

Karl: You see I think Gordon was always very approachable, even when he was playing chess or whatever.

Keith: Yeah but you can say that, because you went to university with him. You lived with him.

Gordon: In the last five years you have all normalized life for me. You've got to understand that.

Stanton: But we've done nothing different, maybe your perception is different?

Gordon: But you see, I didn't have that before in my life here!

Jerome: Did any of you ever see Gordon when he was really ill? Did any of you ever visit him in hospital?

Gordon: My friend Eric was the only one who saw me. In terms of my definition of coping with your illness, the dominoes have allowed me to have a meaningful life.

Stanton: But to be fair, you've allowed that to happen. I don't want to take any accolades for what you call 'recovery' because you've done it yourself.

Gordon: Yeah, but you see you need people around you who will contribute towards your recovery.

Stanton: But you say the 'people around you.' Is it not that you've allowed them to be around you?

Karl: No, it's not like that. It's what is around you...for a lot of people getting back into work is a massive boost for fighting depression.

Gordon: But, listen, it's taken a long time to get to full recovery, many

years – and it's been a lot of hard work – and you've made that work easier.
Karl: I wouldn't say you're yet fully recovered, because you'll be fully recovered when you can get a job and you can go out.

Stanton: Yeah but you see I believe that Gordon's illness has helped him to become what he's always wanted to be in terms of helping people. His contribution to the mental recovery programme is pioneering stuff. Very few people before Gordon have embarked on this journey and, as the title of the book suggests, it's 'one man's march.' It's all him. I don't feel I've had any influence over Gordon – if he turns round and says that I've helped him, well then nice one, but he's allowed me to do that. He could have turned around and said that the dominoes were not doing anything for him – even if they were for us. It's a choice that he's made and it's because his perception and outlook on life has changed. I see Gordon a lot during the week. We'll just reason, we'll sit there and we'll talk and many times we'll be discussing a subject and Gordon will say 'ahhh I didn't see it like that.' He'll see something but he won't see what I saw. How you perceive yourself is the important thing.

Karl: It's also a question of age, you know, because you mellow with age.

Stanton: Through his illness, he's got an outlet now. He's got a website, he's on the verge of publishing a book.

Gordon: That's why you are a very important person. Out of all the people here, Stanton is the most important because he did the website for me. Stanton gave me something to cling on to. He comes every month and he does the website. It gives me something to look forward to – that regularity. The regularity is very important for me: every two weeks I know there is a dominoes session. I prepare my mind for that, so I tell myself 'I don't want to be affected by my illness on Thursday.' And there are days when I don't want to cook and I am depressed, I am hearing voices, I just don't want to know and yet I say to myself 'I have just got to do it, I've got to overcome it.' In that sense it's changed me. You don't know what it's like for me. It gave me something to focus on.

Karl: That's a very good point, because often people find doing things for themselves very difficult but when they have to do them for someone else it's a lot easier.

Karl: One of the good things about the website is that whereas before Gordon would argue his point of view and try to persuade others of it, with the website he can just get his ideas out there.

Gordon: It gives meaning to my life, playing dominoes gives meaning to my life, seeing Stanton and Keith and Karl gives meaning to my life – instead of just getting lost in the schizophrenia and waking up at 4.30/5 o'clock in the morning hearing voices. I can tell you -- that is heavy and it goes on and on. You can't sleep, you have to get up. You have to get up, come in to the front room, turn on the television and distract yourself. You have to. And that is a discipline. You have to learn to cope with your illness. That's why Dr Roberts said that it is often hard work, because you've got to be disciplined, otherwise you are lying in bed listening to the 'voices,' and talking to them. And they will go on until 7 or 8 o'clock. I know because I've tried it.

Stanton: When you hear the 'voices' what is your initial response? Is it anger?

Gordon: Frustration. Why is it happening to me? Why can't it stop? Why can't I just be a normal person?

Karl: You've got to accept them in your life, Gordon.

Gordon: Yeah, in order to be able to cope with it. One part of my definition of recovery is coping with your illness. You've got to cope with it.

Keith: Have you got to cope with it or have you got to beat it?

Gordon: Beat it. That's what I've got to do.

Jerome: One thing that Gordon has done is to bring his intellectual capacities to bear on this concept of recovery, and this concept that he has come up with is so simple yet so comprehensive. There are men and women with many more letters after their name than Gordon, and yet he's given us perhaps the best definition of what recovery is. And he has given lectures and really come out about his illness, which so many people don't do. Families don't do that even, they sometimes want to cover it up.

Gordon: You have to come out about it, you absolutely have to...otherwise people don't know what's going on.

Stanton: It's the stigma that's attached. You know some people feel ashamed and wonder whether they are going to be outcast.

Gordon: That's why it's so important that when I told you guys you didn't outcast me.

Stanton: If you give Gordon something to do he takes it to the next level. It shows in his cooking, in his dominoes and chess. He writes books, he writes articles, and where I believe he has a lack of self-confidence that can also hinder the recovery process. He tends to ask himself questions when he knows the answer deep down.

Karl: That's what I mean about having the passion but still needing the support structure around you.

Gordon: You are all part of my support structure; that's why in the last five years I've felt better. I had to make a choice about telling Dr Carson about the dominoes.

Stanton: Why did you have to make a choice?

Gordon: Because I like to keep things to myself.

Stanton: It's ironic that you feel that way but that you're writing a book, for the world to see.

Gordon: But I don't see myself as writing a book.

Stanton: You're writing a book, yeah, about your journey, about your mental recovery. This book will be published. It will be read by service users and doctors alike. Doctors will learn from it, service users will learn from it. There are a massive constituency of people who need a support structure out there. You've taken your illness and become part of that support system.

Keith: But that's only Gordon being himself!

Stanton: Exactly, that's what I'm trying to get across! He doesn't realize that what he dismisses as simple is actually a major work.

Keith: Exactly, that's what he does...and it may be part of his recovery, but it's more part of his re-finding than his recovery.

Karl: It also takes a very brave person to do that.

Keith: It does, and a smart person -- and one who has the application. And he has all those things. I couldn't do that.

Keith: There are differences too. I've noticed in the last few years that you find it easier to talk about the things in life that your commitments have cost you, which is a big burden for anyone to carry. You know you took up the political causes more than you took on a woman, and you know you gave up a lot for that cause. Before it was anger and it comes out a little bit now still, but at least you will talk about it.

Stanton: It comes down to Gordon being more comfortable letting people into his life and sharing information that is deeply personal to him.

Karl: Also that he's a lot more able now to talk about his illness.

Stanton: Being able to talk about the illness is stage two of the recovery process because in order to do that you need to be able to talk about stage one, which is the acceptance stage. There's a lot of pressure in life to conform to what is considered a normal life. We don't mean to be judgemental but we are, and we do it every day...and on top of all that, you're ill and you've got to cope with that too. That answers the question of why you would hide something like that, because you've got a preconceived idea of how society will deal with you. So acceptance and talking about it are massive steps.

Jerome: The judgements that people make – not when you've got the flu or a broken leg -- but when you say you've got schizophrenia are the 'mother' of all judgements. People suffer terrible discrimination. When Gordon is with you he is accepted, he is one of the lads. In coming out and telling his story, he is telling the story of untold millions who are too afraid to tell. Any final thoughts on what you have learnt from Gordon? Where he could go from here?

Karl: I feel he could move forwards by getting out and about more, maybe playing in some chess tournaments.

Keith: It would be a really rewarding move too.

Karl: Also coping strategies are important, because you'll always be out there and you'll find someone hostile and you've got to develop the social skills to cope with things like that.

Keith: I think it wouldn't be a bad thing for Gordon to fill up a bit more of his time with activity outside the house, anything – just activity outside the house, to fill a little bit more of the space in his mind. Something to give the 'voices' less room to come in. I think it would be good for you to understand the quality of your own self as a person, just give yourself more of a chance.

Gordon: It's hard work though.

Keith: I'm not saying this is something you have to do tomorrow, take it in steps in the future. You'll get bad days of course but you'll start being able to cope with those because you've coped with the bad days in the last five years.

Stanton: I don't really want to make any comments with regards to what Gordon should and shouldn't do from this day forward. I just want to let him know that I've known him for the shortest amount of time, but I was brought up by my Mum in a family that was predominantly female. My Dad was never around. I didn't really have much contact with male role models at all. I felt I got that from The Studio and I felt I definitely got that from being around Gordon and from being part of this domino group. I see Gordon as a big brother. We've become very close. I've got a lot of admiration for him. He's inspired me to do things that I haven't thought I could do before. I've always been into music, I like deejaying but his achievements in the last couple of years have made me wake up and do more things with my life – and it's working. I'm becoming quite successful with what I do, I'm happy with what I do. Gordon has played a big part in that, whether he knows it or not.

Karl pointed out earlier on that he's a great teacher and he is, he's taught me a lot – about his condition, about himself, his politics, his view of the world; and I have learnt and grown from the knowledge that I have received from Gordon directly. Gordon doesn't realize how much he's helped me in the past. I've had family issues, and money problems, and woman problems. Despite him having his own issues he's always been there for me. No questions, no qualms. He wouldn't even think about it for one second. So I mean I love the guy a lot, I've got a lot of affection for him; I'd do anything for him. I will be there on that day when he is officially declared recovered and I know that day is not too far away. And we act in a manner that will bring that day closer as friends and as a support network also.

Eric Ayalande Johnson: A longstanding friend

I was pleasantly surprised and honoured when my friend Gordon asked me to write a little piece about schizophrenia based upon the experiences I have encountered during our friendship. I will start by saying that Gordon has known me even before I was born, when I was a tadpole in my father's loins.

My earliest memory of Gordon was when I was a child of ten years old. He came to my house to visit my father, upon this visit he taught me the rudiments of chess which I thoroughly enjoyed. Occasionally, Gordon would visit my father 3 or 4 times a year at our family home. I would often think to myself, who is this man that would come to the house early in the morning and awake my father? I came to the conclusion that he and my father must be close because my father rarely had visitors to our family home and those that did were wise enough not to come early in the morning. In fact, Gordon and my father have been friends since the 1960s because they both frequented the same school and maintained their friendship till this day. Gordon is one of the few people on this earth that my father truly trusts and respects.

As I grew older, Gordon disappeared off the scene and then re-emerged about ten years later sitting in what used to be up to that moment my chair at work. You see, my father had replaced my services with that of Gordon. I wasn't really angry when I turned up at work to find I was replaced by Gordon. My father was away touring and needed someone he could trust to manage his affairs. I used to do this for him but he sacked me on a number of occasions, and I think I walked out once over an argument about religion. While Gordon was in charge of the office, I used to visit him to frequently to make sure things were running smoothly. During this time I got to know Gordon on a much more personal level and chess was a factor that drew us together. Gordon is an excellent chess player and he agreed to teach me the game seriously because I had developed the chess bug. As our friendship grew I would visit him at his home and we would play chess until the early hours of the morning. Gordon also helped me to smooth out the rough edges of the first poem that I ever wrote which was subsequently printed in a book called 'A Child's Eye View', sponsored by the Millennium Commission. It is a testament to Gordon's character that at this time he was suffering from schizophrenia and I did not have a clue that he was.

My first unconscious experience of Gordon's illness was a time when I said something that he didn't take too kindly to, then Gordon took out a knife and started to wave it frantically all over the place. I was momentarily concerned but my fears were allayed when I asked myself the serious question – 'Would Gordon harm me?' – and I came to the conclusion that answer was simply no. On another occasion I came to visit him, and I pressed his intercom buzzer and looked out of the window and he told me to fuck off. I just went away wondering what I had done to offend him. Gordon is normally a very mild mannered individual; courtesy was and is his broach.

On another occasion I had telephoned him and upon hearing my voice he put the phone down. I still did not know that he was ill at this time.

The real key to me understanding that Gordon was not well was the fact that we both used to frequent a social club, The Studio, where many people of all races and ages would chill-out together. Gordon was always one of the most popular members. This is because many people respected Gordon for his intellect, generosity of spirit and general sunny disposition. However, when the illness was taking root, Gordon would attend this social club and not talk to a single soul, including myself. On another occasion he brought a knife to this club and was told politely to leave the premises, as long as he had that weapon on him, he was not welcome. Soon after this time I did not speak to Gordon apart from the unreturned greetings whenever I saw him. At some point he recognised he was ill and sought medical attention. I think there was period of about 2 years when we didn't speak. I even got married and Gordon who I considered at the time a good friend did not come. This should indicate how much of a recluse he had become or how much the illness had overtaken him. After this 2 year gap Gordon suddenly arrived back from the wilderness to give me a call. He explained to me that he had been suffering from schizophrenia, but was being treated for it. He apologised for his 'alter ego's' bad behaviour and we resumed our friendship. Gordon seemed to be recovering well, then for some reason 1 or 2 years later the illness returned to haunt him. However by this point in time I had become more accustomed to the behavioural symptoms and could tell when Gordon was taking a turn for the worst. He would become a lot more cynical, verbally aggressive and the tone of his voice would become more and more angry by the day/week. In fact I had grown so accustomed to the symptoms that just before Gordon had his last major episode of schizophrenia, I tried to get in contact with his sister Laura, who is a nurse, so she could take the appropriate action. However, I had visited her house only once and could not remember the door number even though I tried by knocking on every door in close proximity. Subsequently I saw Gordon's niece around this time and she gave me Laura's phone number. When I contacted Laura to tell her about Gordon's deterioration she kindly informed me that she already knew and that Gordon had been detained under the Mental Health Act. Soon afterwards Gordon was released. Since being released for the second time Gordon has not been sectioned since.

He has made giant strides in progress but it is deeply upsetting to hear him tell me that he still hears 'voices' but not as much. The 'voices' stop him from sleeping peacefully. The only thing that quiets them down is 2 or 3 bottles of Guinness. Maybe schizophrenia is alcoholic.

Gordon would like to resume his former life as it was before the illness. He used to be a teacher. The stumbling block to him being fully integrated is that he is not fully recovered. He still hears 'voices.' I suggested to him that the medication he is taking is not doing its job and maybe he should try another. He is in agreement but he is afraid of the side-effects of a previously untried medication. He is also scared that the medication might not work and he might suffer a further relapse. He is terrified of being sectioned again and who can blame him? It must be and I am sure it is, a living hell trying to cope with this illness. I personally think he and his psychiatrist should discuss alternative medication at length.

So to conclude: What do I know about schizophrenia?

According to the Penguin English Dictionary, schizophrenia is a mental disorder characterised by loss of contact with reality and disintegration of the personality. My scientific understanding of the matter is basically the brain has difficulty in addressing catastrophic emotional disturbances. The failure of the brain to deal with a big emotional scar or the turning upside down of someone's view of the world brings about unresolved issues that the sub-conscious tries to address by talking to the conscious part of the brain. However, I feel that if one addresses this emotional turbulence and gets to the root of it, the problem can be resolved without the aid of ingested medication.

For me, Gordon is very much in touch with reality and despite his illness his personality is still pretty much the same. On the other hand, I would say that Gordon used to be an extrovert but now he is introverted. He hardly leaves his home. Still, he has a group of friends that visit him fortnightly to play dominoes. These friends are the same people that he met at the social club and he later shunned during his illness. The fact they have continued their friendship says a lot about his place in society and that educated individuals have a good understanding of schizophrenia and its symptoms. However, I would say that the wider community still does not understand the disease. When people have a physical ailment no one looks at it badly, but the moment someone is ill in the head, they tend to shun the individual that is suffering from that disease. Is the human body not one complete organ? I look forward to the day when schizophrenia or its victims are no longer ostracised by the community. Notwithstanding, I do recognise that some sufferers can be a danger to the public and themselves. However, the signs are there and take time to gain momentum. If one is familiar with a sufferer they should be able to see that the individual concerned is about to be consumed and they should then take the appropriate action. This should be done in two stages: ask the person if they are okay, (anger or depression can be misconstrued as schizophrenia), ask them if they are still taking their medicine, if symptoms persists, then medical attention should be sought. That is the GP.

Schizophrenia – this disease has robbed humanity of a brilliant mind and generous soul. However, Gordon's light still burns brightly but could burn even brighter. Gordon doesn't seem to truly recognise this. Gordon taught me chess, helped me with poems, and taught me the concepts of concentration, centralisation, industrial labour force and organic growth, (Editorial comment – Eric is talking about the four features of the General Law of Capitalist Accumulation discovered by Karl Marx) principles all needed to understand what is going on in today's global world. Gordon helped my mother when she decided to do a degree in her forties. He also helped another lady from the social club to obtain a Diploma. Just think what more could Gordon offer to the world if he was 100 per cent? I look forward confidently to the day that Gordon will make a full recovery and take his place in society with the other stars.

Gloria Giraud: Gordon's sister

I am delighted and honoured to have been asked to make a small contribution about the experience and impact Gordon's illness has had upon the family. My recollection of my brother Gordon goes back to our childhood days in Rangoon, Burma, when he was eight years old and his love of reading. He would read anything he could lay his hands on, ie. Mother's womens' magazines imported from the UK, newspapers, the Book of Knowledge, fiction etc. So it comes as no surprise to any of us his interest and enthusiasm with books.

When we first became aware of Gordon's illness 15 years ago, we were totally surprised and could not believe it. I remember saying to our parents when he used to say to us that certain things were happening to him and we thought he was probably 'imagining' it and simply left him to it. We knew that Gordon was actively involved in a number of organisations and played a very active role politically and thought that perhaps someone was jealous of him and wanted him out of the way. So his life continued with no medical help and the years went by without seeing a doctor or medication, until one day when an incident occurred and he was taken to hospital, assessed, then sectioned. It was a very BIG shock to us when he was diagnosed with SCHIZOPHRENIA! How is that possible? It must be DEPRESSION surely and not that word! We were all in denial as it was difficult to accept it. It was indeed the beginning of a very difficult and long road for Gordon.

It was very sad to see him deteriorating like that, as that was NOT the Gordon that we all knew and loved, in our own individual way. It was, indeed, a terrible shock to the whole family. We simply couldn't understand it. We thought that this was due to the numerous disappointments in his personal life and also in his academic career. We all knew that Gordon was a staunch believer in Politics and Communism. His 'so-called' friends gave him no support and had let him down badly. He became 'isolated' for a long time. It must have been terrible for him as we all got on with our own lives.

Today after many years of battling to deal with his many demons, there is a bright light at the end of that very long tunnel. This is due to the continued support of the clinical team, my sister Laura (the nurse in the family) and from Gordon himself, through his own perseverance and determination, has pulled through. I am indeed very happy to see that he is at last been given the recognition he deserves for his writings and intelligence through his publications and his website and monthly writings. I wish him every success with the impending publication of the book written not only by Gordon and Dr Carson, but also contributions from many others. Here's hoping there will be many more to come Gordon. Congratulations on the success of your website and the regular articles you write with sheer conviction and heartfelt dedication. I am very proud of you and so are my daughters Jennifer, Caroline and Annabel Giraud. They remember vividly that Uncle Gordon was humble, gentle in his mannerisms, patient, kind and understanding, always willing to listen and gave sound advice and of course, his laughter was very unusual and distinctive and it amused us all!

6

Jerome on Gordon

Jerome Carson

In this chapter Jerome summarises the themes that emerged over the first three years of his work with Gordon. While they did not know it at the time, Jerome and Gordon were co-developing a recovery approach in practice. Developing a model that explained Gordon's own recovery journey proved very helpful and led to Gordon giving several presentations of his own story of recovery. Gordon was helped by a number of factors, the first of which was his own determination to win his own battle. Other coping strategies that Gordon developed or utilised included the use of writing, chess, dominoes, the recovery literature, the support of family and friends, medication and other therapies such as a hearing 'voices' group in addition to fortnightly sessions with Jerome. While Gordon had hoped to be a communist revolutionary, as Jerome suggests he ended up becoming a mental health revolutionary. The transcript of his comments in Michelle McNary's Recovery Film, confirm this message. As Gordon states, his recovery has been a long and protracted struggle and yet is has been a battle that he was always determined to win. The publication of this book shows he has.

Introduction

In this chapter I summarise some of the main issues arising from the work that I did with Gordon from when I first saw him in January 2007 to December 2009, when we did the bulk of our recovery work together. In fact we continued to meet once a fortnight until August 2011, when I retired from the Health Service. I have tried to arrange the content of our work under themes, to give the reader a sense of how Gordon perceived many of the key issues in his recovery journey. I have also put the date when Gordon raised specific issues from my individual session notes, to try and give a sense of the chronology and development in his thinking over time.

As was mentioned in the Introductory chapter, Gordon was referred to me by Simon Gent, his community psychiatric nurse and care co-ordinator at the time. Gordon had finished his six months of cognitive behaviour therapy at the PICuP Clinic at the Maudsley Hospital. Apart from feeling that Gordon was going through a post therapy depression, I think Simon also felt that Gordon would benefit from the opportunity to talk over many of the issues that were not addressed in his therapy, which was focussed more on the problem with his 'voices'.

Gordon's problems

The first three times I saw Gordon, the assessment interviews were conducted by Dr Laura Southgate, who was one of my clinical trainees at that time. Laura conducted the sessions while I took notes. At one of our earlier meetings, Gordon stated, 'I don't know what life holds for me, apart from schizophrenia and depression,' (20/2/07). Depression was something that Gordon complained of quite a bit. Depression is often a feature in the lives of people with long term psychosis, but the focus of psychological therapy tends to be more geared to delusions and hallucinations, rather than the accompanying depression. 'I've been depressed since I last saw you,' (17/4/07). The other issue that troubled Gordon was emphysema. 'I can't see myself lasting for another four or five years,' (19/3/07). 'I'm too physically ill with emphysema, I couldn't work again,' (27/7/07).

An ordinary life?

Even for professionals who spend their entire careers working with people with long term mental health problems, it can be hard to appreciate the nature of their patients' daily struggles. Gordon put it like this, 'There have been very few days of my life that I can say have been good days for me,' (20/2/07). 'Today's a good day. I got up at 5.00am. It's the first time this year, I feel happy coming for a therapy session,' (18/10/07). On another occasion he commented, 'I went to the pub on Sunday evening. This was the first time I'd been to the pub for six years,' (27/4/09). When we had our first ever service user Oscar's ceremony, Gordon said it was the first time in seven years that he had put on a shirt and tie, (17/12/09).

The effects of mental illness on Gordon

As he points out in his chapters, Gordon had four hospital admissions, in 1994, 1995, 2000 and 2002/3. He said prior to developing schizophrenia, 'I had no problems. I had a fulfilled life, with teaching, chess and socialising,' (18/5/07). 'After my last admission, it took two years to get back together. It's like you have to start all over again,' (30/5/07). He claimed that the illness, 'had broken me down. I became non co-operative, negative and distrustful of people,' (2/4/07). 'I'm reclusive, so I don't get too entangled with other people. If I see more people, I hallucinate about them,' (12/7/07). He also commented that living with the illness was like a battle. 'Nothing prepares you for the battle with mental illness,' (26/7/07) and again, 'This is the biggest battle of my life and I don't intend to lose it,' (28/5/09).

The prospect of future employment

In Chapter 12, Rachel Perkins, one of Gordon's heroes, talks about the importance of work in recovery. Gordon taught business studies for 12 years, but had to give up work due to ill health in 1992. This was a source of great regret. 'I do mourn the fact I lost a teaching career,' (2/4/07), and yet 20 months later Gordon commented, 'The government wants us to go back to work, yet it takes me two to three hours to write a page,'(10/12/08). So while Gordon misses his teaching career, he feels that his problems are such that he would be unable to return to full-time employment.

The mental health services

Gordon has had prolonged contact with mental health services, since the early 1990s. He believed that most of his early illness career was dominated by a medical model of care, with little individual attention to his needs. Indeed he was actually discharged from the service in 1999 and broke down and was readmitted to hospital the following year. 'When they put me into Recovery and Support, there was no recovery plan, only a Care Programme Approach,' (CPA) (24/1/08). 'CPA monitors your illness, not your recovery,' (31/1/08). Despite some of the problems and shortcomings in his care, Gordon still feels very indebted to the local mental health service. His involvement with the recovery work meant, 'I am contributing back something to a service that has looked after me for the last 15 years,' (27/4/09).

Communism

In Chapter 1, Gordon outlined his involvement with communist politics in Britain. It was clearly a very difficult period for him and he mentioned this numerous times in our sessions. The following quotations give some flavour of his thinking. 'I gave everything to politics,' (23/1/07). 'I was the hard man of the communist movement. I had value then,' (18/5/08). He felt that his teaching was only a means to supplement his political activities. '1980/81 was a traumatic period. It was the first communist organisation I joined, but I was expelled within a year. Comradeship went out the window at times,' (30/10/08). 'I was the top communist philosopher of my generation. I knew dialectics, empiricism, classical German philosophy,' (19/2/09).

Living with the 'voices'

Amongst the most distressing symptoms experienced by people with schizophrenia are auditory and visual hallucinations, so-called positive symptoms. Negative symptoms of the illness relate to apathy, lack of energy and motivation. Gordon still continued to experience distressing 'voices' despite being on fortnightly neuroleptic depot injections, which he received at the community teambase. He was normally wakened by the 'voices' each day at 4.00 or 5.00am. 'The 'voices" go at you. It's like the radio gets turned on and you can't turn it off,' (23/1/07). This would often mean he would get little sleep at nights and would be exhausted trying to keep everything together. 'There are days when the 'voices" get at you and you don't eat for two or three days. All I do is smoke and drink coffee,' (13/6/07). 'I'm frightened to write about the 'voices". That's why I write in a very general way. I'm trying to objectify my condition, and not get lost in it,' (13/6/07). One of the ways he copes is by having BBC News 24 on all day to distract him. 'I compared myself to John Nash,' (9/8/07). 'I learned the lesson from **A Beautiful Mind.** Ignore the 'voices." Distract yourself. Keep yourself busy, so I don't get caught up in the 'voices',' (18/10/07). He finds nighttimes the hardest period and has found he can generally only get off to sleep if he has a couple of bottles of Guinness. It would often strike me, as I would also be getting up at around 4.30am to get ready for work, that Gordon would already be up. Unlike me though, he was being tormented by his 'voices'. In fact I would sometimes call him at around 8.00am, knowing he would already have been up for a few hours.

Thoughts on recovery

'There are those of us who want to recover. In 2001, I resolved to do something about my life. I did not have a specific recovery plan,' (24/1/08). 'I've lost 14 years. You have to cope first. Then you have to have hope,' (14/2/08). Seven months later he came up with his definition of recovery, **'It's coping with your illness and trying to have a meaningful life,'** (18/9/08). This very succinct definition, may well be one of his greatest contributions to the field of recovery. It suggests that each individual has to be able to cope with the unique pattern of symptoms that their mental illness entails. They also have to try and find a life for themselves that is imbued with meaning. Gordon cautions, 'Recovery is a protracted process. It's a tough struggle,' (15/10/09). He also commented that, 'We can be experts by experience when we are in the recovery stage, not when we are acutely ill,' (27/4/09).

Gordon's model of recovery

Gordon talks about his model in Chapter 3. He has also been interested in the notion of rationality and irrationality. Recovery means moving from a state of irrational thinking, when the individual is psychotic, to a process of more rational thinking. 'It didn't come to me in two months. It took nearly a year in therapy,' (24/1/08). His five stage model of his own recovery was not fully articulated until the middle of January 2008. It starts with a normal pre-illness phase. Then his hospital breakdown. This is followed by his period of deep schizophrenia. The fourth stage is a stage of recovery. The last stage is the resumption of a normal life. 'I look at the model and I can see I've come a long way,' (30/6/09).

The first presentation

In October 2007, we had the first presentation at our new Recovery Group (Morgan and Carson, 2009). We had previously had a monthly user group (see Chapter 7). The idea of our new Recovery Group was to have inspiring presentations from people who used our services, which might encourage others in their own journeys of recovery. As his therapist and also the organiser of the Recovery Group, I could see that Gordon would be a really good presenter. In sessions, I began to float the idea of Gordon presenting at one of the group's meetings. His initial positive response was slowly dissipating at the date of his presentation came closer, 'I don't feel I'm ready for it yet. I don't know if I want to come out,' (10/1/08). Working on his own individual model helped change his mind. I suggested that I could simply interview him in front of the audience and we would just go over the model we had developed. While we had to put the presentation date back by two weeks, within this period he changed his mind, 'I feel I can now make the presentation,' (24/1/08). His sister came along to hear the presentation, and indeed Gordon agreed for his sister's boyfriend to film the interview. There were over 20 people present at the teambase that day, including several staff. Gordon claimed that he was 'shattered' by the presentation, and indeed that it took him four or five days to recover from it. His sister was delighted and commented she had not seen him like that for years. Gordon stated, 'I've never talked about my life to complete strangers. Charlene was the only member of staff present who had seen me at my worst between 2001-2003.' Not only did Gordon inspire the service users that day, it was the first time that staff had heard a service user articulate a vision of their own recovery. I told Gordon I felt it was a 'tour de force,' and that 'he had given me one of the best days of my life.' Indeed I rang my wife after his presentation and asked her to put a bottle of white wine in the fridge so I could celebrate when I got back from work!

Gordon's goals

The issue of goals is something that Gordon has thought of from his very first session in January 2007. 'My first task is not to be in hospital. I'm here to recover, second goal.' The fact that he had achieved goals in the past led to this puzzlement. 'I achieved my goals. I became a teacher. I became a communist leader. I achieved my chess goals. I don't understand why I broke down!' (26/7/07). By June of that year, he changed his goals slightly to not being hospitalised, managing and coping with 'voices' and his third goal was to recover. In November of that year, he felt his greatest achievement was that he had not had a breakdown in the last two years. The following July he had expanded his goals to four. Avoid a breakdown. Control my symptoms. Hope for recovery. To give life meaning. This is also something he touches on in Michelle McNary's Recovery Film, which I will mention later.

Writing as a coping strategy

Gordon has used writing as a coping strategy for many years. The first major writing task he set himself when he resolved to try and change his situation in 2001, was to try and write a book on globalisation. 'I wrote the Globalisation book to get rid of the schizophrenia, which I did not succeed in doing,' (13/6/07). 'I began the book on Globalisation in 2001, after a friend had asked me for a Marxist explanation of Globalisation. This took four years to complete,' (17/1/08). Another friend set up a website for Gordon (www.globalmessenger.cjb.net). He posts a monthly newsletter on this with his views on any political topic that has attracted his attention. Thus far over 400 people have visited his website. Gordon has also written more on the topic of recovery over recent years, see McManus (2008), McManus et al (2009), Carson, McManus and Chander (2010), McManus (2011). He also featured in the Psychosis Stories of Recovery and Hope book, (Cordle et al, 2011).

Chess as a coping strategy

Chess has always been very important to Gordon. He talks about teaching people chess in The Studio. 'I was a chess enthusiast. I was the Battersea Handicap Champion,' (2/4/07). 'I met Kasparov and Karpov (previous world chess champions) in the past,' (2/4/07). Yet, 'Everytime I break down, I lose the ability to play chess. That's why I play chess as a means of recovery,' (18/10/07). 'Chess is an outlet that is helping me recover, yet I am still hearing 'voices" about it,' (10/6/08). 'I'm using chess to try and ignore the 'voices'.' Undoubtedly a major step forward with both this writing and his chess, was when his sister Moira gave him a computer. This meant he could search the Internet for material for his book on Globalisation. It also meant that he could purchase a computer programme, to enable him to play chess against the computer programme. Gordon has thought about rejoining a chess club. He entered an open chess competition last year and managed to play several games over a two day period, despite his ongoing and enduring symptoms.

The dominoes group

In Chapter 5, the current dominoes group were interviewed by Sophie Davies and myself. Gordon talked about playing dominoes at The Studio. After The Studio closed in 2004, Gordon offered to host the dominoes playing in his flat. Once a fortnight, Keith, Karl and Stanton come to Gordon's. He generally cooks them a curry and they settle down to an evening of dominoes and drinking. Being a part of this group has been hugely important to Gordon in his recovery. The group have also been able to share and celebrate his recovery successes. Indeed his friend Keith came along to see him receive his Oscar for his writings on recovery.

Family and friends

As stated above, the dominoes crew have been very important in keeping Gordon involved in the wider social world outside of mental health services. These friends 'have kept faith in me,' (20/2/07). 'I told a friend I was schizophrenic. I am coming out to my friends,' (18/10/07). His sister Laura has been his 'carer' for many years. While this was a positive, it was also a worry at times, 'She'll get me put into hospital if I start behaving irrationally,' (13/6/07). I reassured Gordon on this point. His sister also encouraged him to use cleaning as a type of therapy and reminded him to make sure he was always properly dressed. Gordon is also in regular contact with his mother, now in her nineties. Indeed he calls her every morning.

Influences from the wider recovery movement

Gordon has been influenced by five main writers on the subject of recovery and coping with schizophrenia. One of the first writers I introduced Gordon to, was Patricia Deegan (Deegan, 1996). 'Deegan suffered schizophrenia from a young age. She went through the system 35 years ago. She had a goal to become a psychologist. In the process she fought against the system. I saw her as a revolutionary,' (26/7/07). Later he commented, 'I couldn't relate to Deegan at first. It took me six months. She had her own battle. She became an insider to do it,' (31/1/08). One of the things we did together was to watch a video of Patricia Deegan delivering the 1996 paper at a conference in Rotterdam. As Gordon watched this, I made notes, on how I felt her message related to his own journey of recovery, which I later typed up for him. A second influence was James Bellamy (Bellamy, 2000). James wrote an account of his own experience of psychosis, which moved Gordon. 'James Bellamy fascinated me. He talked of visual hallucinations. I talk about forms,' (13/06/07). Talking of both he noted, 'People like Deegan and Bellamy have made me aware of other people with schizophrenia,' (13/06/07). Reading or listening to someone's accounts of their illness must be so reassuring to many sufferers, as these experiences are often outside the knowledge of most families. When Joel Slack asked his father to help him when he was experiencing psychosis, his father replied, 'Son, I don't know how to help you!'

Rachel Perkins is another person who has influenced Gordon. I had given Gordon a copy of her book chapter, 'You need hope to cope,' (Perkins, 2006). Gordon said, 'I found it the most relevant to understanding what recovery is, even though I don't fully understand recovery yet,' (13/6/07). Gordon has also read quite a bit of the work of Peter Chadwick (see Chapters 8 and 9), and attended the Recovery Group session when Peter came down to Streatham. Dolly Sen is another of his heroes though Gordon found it very difficult reading the first book of her autobiography (Sen, 2002). He commented, 'I'm using these articles to develop my analytical approach, which I lost during my period of schizophrenia,' (11/2/09). Providing Gordon with these articles made him 'feel like a student getting handouts,' (28/6/07), yet as he said he went through all the handouts now and then and 'read them to keep me going,' (3/4/08).

The idea of a book on recovery?

At the first ever session with Gordon he mentioned that he was thinking about 'writing a book on schizophrenia,' (23/1/07). It was in November of that year that I mentioned a title of 'From Communism to Schizophrenia.'

At the end of March 2008, I suggested we write a book together. His response the following month was, 'I'm not interested in the money. I'm surprised a book could be in the making.' In July, when we heard that the book proposal had been accepted he stated, 'My view is that I want two things. Mental health professionals should have a better understanding of what recovery means. Second, I want the patients to see there is hope of recovery.'

Other therapies

In addition to seeing me once a fortnight, Gordon also attended a hearing 'voices' group, which was one of his first encounters with other voice hearers. Prior to seeing me, he had six months of cognitive behaviour therapy. 'My CBT therapist treated schizophrenia like cancer,' (15/11/07). 'They taught me to cope. You are teaching me to think,' (17/4/07). Gordon, after some hesitation, decided to come along to a one day self-esteem workshop (Carson, 2006). This proved very helpful for him, especially as he received such positive feedback from other members at the workshop. One said he was 'highly intellectual but very humble' and another that he was 'inspirational.' Gordon also completed a short programme of Acceptance and Commitment Therapy (ACT) with Eric Morris, one of my senior psychology colleagues, which he also found beneficial.

Jerome with Gordon

In reading through the individual session notes, apart from writing down a lot of what Gordon said in sessions, I sometimes wrote down points I wanted to stress to Gordon.'My task is to help you see the value in yourself as a person and the contribution you are making and can make,' (19/3/07). 'Your model is a road map for your recovery,' (24/1/08). 'You are one of the most remarkable patients I have ever met. You have taught me so much,' (6/2/08). 'Ask yourself, what have I gained, not what have I lost?' (22/5/05). 'You are a revolutionary in mental health,' (13/11/08). 'Neither of us could have foreseen that you would go from reading about recovery to writing about it,' (27/7/09).

Contributions to recovery

I mentioned above Gordon' first ever Recovery Group presentation. Since then he presented at a workshop held as part of a recovery training event in Lambeth in May 2009. He also presented to two recovery workshops that we held at the Teambase. The largest audience he faced was over 40 social work masters degree students at Kingston University, when Matt Ward, Gordon and myself did a joint presentation on recovery. Finally, he spoke at the Annual General Meeting of Southside Rehabilitation Association to an audience of staff, workers and trustees. The format for these presentations has remained similar to his first ever teaching session. That is, I take him through his model of recovery. If he comes to a halt, I ask another question to get him going again. He is always remarkably fluent and convincing.

One of his biggest achievements was to agree to participate in Michelle McNary's Recovery Film. While I nominated him for this and he was also keen to help Michelle out, he still had to be auditioned by Dr Paul Wolfson and Michelle. They had no hesitation as soon as they interviewed him. The film brings out the philosopher in Gordon. I have transcribed his comments from the film and they are written below.

Gordon's comments taken from Michelle McNary's Recovery Film

Recovery means that you are looking for a new....*self*, a new meaning, a new identity.

The challenge is to try to have an awareness of....that you are mentally ill. That is the major challenge, that anyone has...to recognise that you are that you are mentally ill and to confront it. That is the biggest challenge. That leads you in my opinion on the road to recovery.

Recovery is a new concept in mental illness and it's not widely practised yet in this country. So we are doing a job trying to develop it, from the patients' point of view...and so the therapy is important that way we express ourselves, where we come to terms with ourselves and where we can try to rebuild our life for ourselves.

I have been lucky, you know, I have been very lucky that my family have looked after me; my friends have been helpful, two or three...even though one says I've got I've a few loose screws, which I can understand.

..and I've got a book on globalisation, you know, which I wrote, which I'm happy with it got rid of the majority of the political 'voices,' I swear to you, because I was having bad experiences and I said to myself if this helps, if this comes out right, I'm on the road to recovery and it came out right and I'm on the road to recovery.

My cause is, I know my cause, I have learned about my cause, my cause is paranoia, leading to disillusionment with the capitalist life in Britain and the negativities that surrounds it and I wasn't positive to those changes. I didn't act in a proper rational way, constructing my life, I went negative over it. During the period of schizophrenia, heavy schizophrenia, you suffer from the lost years and so you're trying to get that back again. So you've lost your personality, you've lost your identity, you've lost your meaning and so you're trying to get it back in your recovery and that's all, that's what you're hoping for, in recovery, to get those things back.

When it's severe the 'voices' just come at me at one hundred miles per hour. You know it's just 'voices' hitting me left, right and centre. I just sit there smoking, drinking coffee and talking to the 'voices.' That could be all day, it could be two or three days.

...and it's a slow protracted process recovery. You know, I had a cold, it went away in a week and I was better but you know recovery from schizophrenia is not like that; it's a long, slow protracted process and you've got to keep at it and you've got to keep positive and have hope, otherwise you're not going to get there.

Well, the immediate goal is to be fully recovered from schizophrenia; that is my immediate goal. If that's a dream, then that's a dream that I hold to. To go back to teaching, even though I'm getting short of years now.

Jerome on Gordon

In his Foreword to the book, Mental Health Recovery Heroes Past and Present, Professor Geoff Shepherd makes the following comments:

.... if staff retained the feeling of excitement and discovery that usually characterises our first meetings with people we have been asked to see. As

Jerome Carson comments when Gordon McManus was referred to his team, Fortunately for me, I was the one asked to see him. I found this simple assertion of values both moving and challenging. This book opens our eyes again to the rich voyages of discovery that we are sometimes privileged to share with the extraordinary people that are described in its pages. I thank the authors for bringing them together and I thank the contributors for sharing their lives,' (Shepherd, 2011, p.7).

I was of course lucky to be the person chosen to see Gordon. As the first half of this book shows, he is a remarkable man, who has always tried to live his life by his principles, from his early days as a student activist. He seemed set on a lifelong career in teaching, combined with his involvement in communist politics. Unfortunately at the age of 39 he began to become mentally unwell. Initially his parents tried to care for him, but in 1994 he was admitted to mental hospital and for the next decade he was to have three further admissions and was diagnosed with paranoid schizophrenia. In 2001 he resolved to try and change his life, but less than two years later he was admitted to hospital for the last time. When I first saw Gordon at the start of 2007, I realised immediately that this was an amazing man, who would be a pleasure to work with. He has been one of the individuals who has helped me to develop my own ideas about recovery, from being sceptical at first. Our work together started before my work with any of the other individuals who were to be so important to the development of recovery. I was also fortunate in having the flexibility to work with Gordon over a much longer period than anyone else had. His CBT therapist worked with him for six months. Some would argue that this was a very cost ineffective way of working. Yet, the work we have done together has led to so much happening for us both, which could only have occurred over a longer time span. Indeed, it took us a year to develop Gordon's model of recovery. Now that I am retired from the NHS, I of course miss our regular sessions, and yet I know Gordon is only a phone call away or I can e-mail him and vice versa. The late great football manager Bill Shankley once said that 'football wasn't a matter of life or death, it was more important than that.' He was of course wrong. At the end of the day football is only a game, albeit a great game. Recovery on the other hand can be a matter of life and death. Hopefully with the leadership and example provided by Gordon and many others, more sufferers will choose to live. Our task as professionals is clear. Following Gordon, we need to help people cope with their illness and have a meaningful life. Recovery can be a protracted process and a tough struggle and possibly the biggest battle of your life, but as Gordon would also say, it is not one that you should intend to lose.

References

Bellamy, J. (2000) Can you hear me thinking? *Psychiatric Rehabilitation Journal,* 24, 1, 73-75

Carson, J. (2006) *Be Your Own Self-Esteem Coach.* London: Whiting and Birch

Carson, J. McManus, G. & Chander, A. (2010) Recovery; a selective review of the literature. *Mental Health and Social Inclusion,* 14, 1, 35-44

Cordle, H. Fradgley, J. Carson, J. Holloway, F. & Richards, P. (2011) *Psychosis Stories of Recovery and Hope.* London: Quay Books

Deegan, P. (1996) Recovery as a journey of the heart. *Psychiatric Rehabilitation Journal,* 19, 3, 91-97

McManus, G. (2008) Gordon's story. In, Carson, J. Holloway, F. Wolfson, P. & McNary, M. London: South London and Maudsley NHS Foundation Trust

McManus, G. Morgan, S. Fradgley, J. & Carson, J. (2009) Recovery heroes- a profile of Gordon McManus. *A Life in the Day,* 13, 4, 16-19

McManus, G. (2011) Gordon McManus. In, Davies, S. Wakely, E. Morgan, S. & Carson, J. (Eds), *Mental Health Recovery Heroes Past and Present.* Brighton: OLM-Pavilion

Morgan, S. & Carson, J. (2009) The recovery group: a service user and professional perspective. *Groupwork,* 19, 1, 26-39

Perkins, R. (2006) You need hope to cope. In, Roberts, G. Davenport, S. Holloway, F. & Tattan, T. (Eds), *Enabling Recovery: The Principles and Practice of Rehabilitation Psychiatry.* London: Gaskell

Sen, D. (2002) *Can You Hear Me Laughing?* Brentwood: Chipmunka Press

Shepherd, G. (2011) Foreword. In, Davies, S. Wakely, E. Morgan, S. & Carson, J. (Eds), *Mental Health Recovery Heroes Past and Present.* Brighton: OLM-Pavilion.

Part Two

Roads to Recovery

7
Recovery from severe mental illness
A personal journey and a look at recovery from top to bottom

Jerome Carson

In this chapter, Jerome looks at four areas. Firstly, he gives an account of his own career in mental health services. Secondly, he looks at the background to the recovery approach. He considers definitions of recovery and some of the published research. His aim is to be illustrative rather than exhaustive. Some of this work, particularly around the issue of policy, could be described as the 'top down' approach to recovery, for example this is how you ought to do it, and the recent Sainsbury Report Making Recovery a Reality *fits into this approach. Thirdly, he looks at a 'bottom-up approach' that has been developed for recovery in the South-West Sector in the Lambeth Directorate of the South London and Maudsley NHS Foundation Trust, where he worked. This looks at a number of small initiatives that are aimed to help individuals with their personal recovery journeys. He discusses the Recovery Group, Recovery Workshops, Recovery Film, Recovery Heroes, Recovery Oscars, and individual recovery work. Finally, he describes what has helped him on this personal recovery journey. This covers the financial support that he has received, the support of international recovery experts, local managerial and clinical support, and the influence of people who use services on his work. It shows how even small local initiatives require assistance from multiple sources if they are to thrive. His own journey as a clinician to understand and work with the recovery approach is parallel to and influenced by the journeys of the people who use our services, especially Gordon, who has inspired the writing of this book.*

Part 1. My personal career in mental health

I often cite the title of the series of discussion papers by the Social Perspectives Network, *Whose Recovery is it Anyway?* It is of course the service users' recovery (Social Perspectives Network, 2007). This reminds us that our focus as professionals needs to be on helping people who use our services towards their own individual recovery. At the time of writing, I am fully committed towards the recovery approach. To tell the reader how I got there, I have to say something of my own background in psychiatry and how the specialism has changed over the years.

From university to asylum

In 1979, I graduated with a degree in psychology from Reading University. During the three year degree course, I realised that I wanted to pursue a career in clinical psychology. There were then comparatively few training places available and intense competition for these. To secure a training place it was necessary to obtain 'relevant experience,' after graduation. The best experience was felt to be getting a job as an assistant psychologist or as it was also referred to in those days, psychology technician. I made a number of unsuccessful applications and in the end was forced to seek work as a nursing assistant. I worked initially at Fairmile Hospital for two months, before moving to a similar post at Borocourt Hospital. I was told that the Mary Sheridan Unit was looking for psychology graduates, who though employed as nursing assistants, would have the opportunity to become involved in clinically based research. Having worked here for a year, I then applied for a training place in clinical psychology. I was only asked along to one interview at Manchester University, and I failed to be offered a place there. What to do next?

From asylum to asylum

I reasoned that two years experience as a nursing assistant would be regarded as not much better than the one year's experience that I already had. I determined to try again to secure one of the coveted assistant psychologist posts. Having the years nursing experience behind me, I now managed to get interviews for assistant jobs. After a number of 'near misses' I was offered a job at Horton Hospital in Epsom, as an assistant psychologist on a Token Economy Research Project.

The Token Economy Ward

Horton Hospital was one of five hospitals located within a square mile on the outskirts of Epsom. The other psychiatric hospitals were Long Grove and West Park. The Manor Hospital and St. Ebba's Hospital, provided services to people with learning disabilities, referred to in those days as the mentally handicapped. In 1980, mental hospitals were in their heyday, though change was coming quicker than staff realised. The project that I was employed to work on, aimed to use a Token Economy system, to improve the functional living skills of patients, who had been resident in mental hospitals for many decades. In brief, patients were given their hospital benefits payments in the form of plastic tokens, which they had to earn for achieving specified behavioural targets. You might receive 10 tokens for making your bed in the morning, 10 for having a shave etc. Tokens could then be exchanged for goods in the ward shop. The most popular purchase was of course cigarettes. Having worked on this project for a year, I eventually achieved my goal of securing a training place.

Clinical psychology training

I arrived to train in clinical psychology at the then North East London Polytechnic in 1981. Eight young psychologists started the three year course, though one dropped out in the first year. Of the eight, only three of us were paid. The other five had to support themselves through the training and pay their own tuition fees. I had been sponsored onto the course by the City and Hackney Health Authority, and was based at Hackney Hospital, not the more glamorous St. Bartholomew's Hospital. At Hackney, the psychiatric unit, 'F Block,' was based in an old workhouse, in the general hospital. These District General Hospital Units (DGHs), were said then to be the future of psychiatry and the main replacement for the old mental hospitals, located as many were, well away from their catchment areas. Horton in Epsom for example, served Kensington and Chelsea.

The Worcester Development Project

When I finished my training in 1984, I then had to find work as a clinical psychologist. Surprisingly at the time, there was no work to be found in London and I had to relocate with my wife and young son to Kidderminster in the West Midlands. In contrast to Hackney, the Kidderminster Unit, based in 'D' Block of the general hospital, was purpose built and modern. Huge amounts of money had been 'pumped into' Kidderminster in an attempt to develop local services to enable the closure of Powick Hospital in Worcester. Like Horton, Powick was a large asylum. By now, governments had decided to close the large asylums. They were seen as representing the worst of psychiatric practice following a number of institutional scandals. It was also assumed that community care might be cheaper. Most of the large asylums were around 100 years old and were becoming expensive to maintain. The so-called DGH model of psychiatry, was felt to be the template for future mental health services, though psychiatry was not always welcomed by general medicine. Interestingly, none of the patients that I saw in Kidderminster had ever been inpatients at Powick Hospital. So it seemed that the psychologists at least, were working with a different population. My wife and I had been unable to sell our own house in London and following a burst pipe and flooding in the cold winter of 1985, we decided to cut our losses and return to London.

Back to the asylum

Returning to London proved easier than leaving it. I now had some post-qualification experience and after a few job interviews, decided to take a post at Claybury Hospital at Woodford Bridge in Essex. I arrived at Claybury in the middle of the closure process. I was recruited to work in the hospital's rehabilitation service, though increasingly also in planning new community services, for when the hospital closed. I spent almost seven years at Claybury. One of the other psychologists at Claybury was Fabian Davis. He was an advocate of the normalisation approach, also known as social role valorisation. This shaped his approach to the resettlement process. The preferred community living arrangement for advocates of this approach, was for patients to live in 'ordinary housing' and to lead 'ordinary lives.' One project in Waltham Forest run by the local MIND organisation, had a number of patients living in small houses on their own, with staff providing peripatetic support. Staff were there to assist patients live their lives, not to run or control their lives as had been the case in the highly regulated asylums. Many patients found this degree of freedom quite difficult to get used to. The Claybury closure was exceptionally well monitored by the Team for the Assessment of Psychiatric Services, who looked at the closure of Friern Barnet and Claybury Hospitals (Leff, 1997). By and large the move to the community was not the disaster that many hospital staff had predicted, and there was undoubtedly an improvement in patients' quality of life, though probably a shrinkage in their social networks. Towards the end of 1991, I decided that I needed a fresh challenge and decided to apply for a post at the Institute of Psychiatry, as a lecturer in psychiatric rehabilitation.

Inner city psychiatry

Part of the reason for leaving Claybury, was the opportunity to work with the consultant psychiatrist, Dr Frank Holloway (see chapter 11 by Harding and Holloway in this book). I had read a number of Frank's book chapters and felt he would be an inspiring psychiatrist to work with. I was not to be disappointed. In April 1992, I arrived to work at St. Giles psychiatric day hospital in Camberwell. Frank had set up the Camberwell Resettlement Team, which had arranged the repatriation of Lambeth residents back to the community from Cane Hill Hospital, in Coulsden, Surrey. Frank and others were involved in designing a new community based mental health service, that included both residential and day care provision. Residential facilities included supported housing schemes, as well as a community hospital hostel, called Townley Road. Day care provision included the setting up of a sheltered work scheme called Southside Rehabilitation Association and a social club called the 48 Club, as well as the established day hospital. When I arrived, Dr Holloway was in the process of setting up a case management service, which like so many initiatives in psychiatry, had been imported from America. Case management was an innovative way of working with patients in the community, involving a more holistic approach to care, which was a precursor of the Care Programme Approach.

From day hospital to community mental health team

In 1995, the then Bethlem and Maudsley NHS Trust decided to reorganise its community services. In East Lambeth this meant establishing two community mental health centres, one in West Norwood, the other in Brixton. Dr Holloway opted to move to Norwood and I moved with him. Unlike the provision in West Lambeth, we established two generic consultant led mental health teams. Shortly after both halves of Lambeth merged in 1999, the Norwood Team divided into an Assessment and Treatment and a Case Management Team, to mirror the provision in the other half of Lambeth. Towards the end of 2005, Lambeth services were re-organised again and the five community mental health teams were reduced from five to three. Dr Peter Hayward and myself had to make a decision as to who worked in Norwood and who moved to Streatham. Peter chose to move to Norwood, which meant I moved to Streatham.

The South-West Sector CMHT and Recovery and Support

In January 2006 I moved to work in the Streatham service. As part of the reconfiguration of services, the case management team was renamed the recovery and support team. As the consultant psychologist for the sector, I was able to work across both teams. This gave me the chance to start reading about the concept of recovery. I decided that it would be helpful to offer the recovery and support team some teaching and one of the earliest sessions I put on was, 'Who put the recovery into recovery and support?' In the early days I was sceptical of the concept of recovery and rather agreed with the approach taken by Whitwell (1999), that recovery was a myth and that survival might be a better concept. I was invited back to the Norwood Team to give them a similar presentation. At the time we had an American social worker in the team called Arnold Kruger. He had only published one professional paper and it was on the topic of recovery (Kruger, 2000). We had a debate in the teambase, with him arguing the case for recovery and me the case against. Slowly and inexorably, I began to change my own views on recovery and now am one of its strongest advocates. It was about this time that I was asked to see a new patient called Gordon McManus. Along with other patients, Gordon has helped shape my own views on recovery.

Part 2: Recovery: The top down approach

What is recovery?

There are of course many definitions of recovery. Arguably one of the most influential has been Professor Bill Anthony's,

> Recovery is a deeply personal, unique process of changing one's attitudes, values, feelings, skills and roles. It is a way of living a satisfying, hopeful and contributing life, even with the limitations caused by illness. Recovery involves the development of new meaning and purpose in one's life as one grows beyond the catastrophic effects of mental illness. (Anthony, 1993)

Jacobson and Greenley define it differently in terms of internal and external conditions. Hence they state,

> ... the word recovery refers to both internal conditions- the attitudes, experiences and processes of change of individuals who are recovering- and external conditions- the circumstances, events, policies and practices that may facilitate recovery. Together internal and external conditions produce the process called recovery. (Jacobson and Greenley, 2001)

In contrast to these definitions of recovery provided by academics, I find myself even more admiring of the definitions offered by people who use mental health services, such as:

+ recovery is longevity in wellbeing (Ajayi et al, 2009, p.34).
+ recovery is an individual journey towards a more valued life (p.35).
+ recovery is about getting things together (p.35).
+ Gordon's own definition fits well with these other service user definitions, 'recovery is coping with your illness and having a meaningful life,' (McManus, 2008).
+ Recovery is an idea whose time has come. (Shepherd et al, 2008).

Unusually it is an idea that is embraced by policy makers, professionals, service users and carers. Yet people like Patricia Deegan were articulating concepts of recovery over two decades ago (Deegan, 1988). Our recent selective review of the recovery literature (Carson et al, 2010), attempted to summarise the top 10 journal papers, the top 10 policy reports, the top 10 books and the top 10 websites on recovery.

The top recovery journal papers

In terms of journal papers, one of the most significant papers was Patricia Deegan's 'recovery as a journey of the heart,' (Deegan, 1996). This paper contains so much helpful and thought provoking material. By the age of 18, Patricia had already been admitted three times to a mental hospital. Yet, amazingly, she embarked on a journey of recovery. While she was training to become a clinical psychologist, she had another admission in her first year, and again she went on to complete her clinical training. Onken et al (2007), call her a recovery visionary. Having watched her video of this talk over 100 times, I feel I know her personally!

The other papers we cited were Whitwell (1999), Andresen et al (2003), Roberts and Wolfson (2004), Davidson et al (2005), Liberman and Kopelowicz (2005), Resnick and Rosenheck (2006), Chadwick (2006), Onken et al (2007) and Warner (2009). Rather than go over each one in detail, I will just select a few and summarise key messages for recovery from each. Whitwell's (1999) paper was quite an influential one for me early in my reading of the literature. He observed that very few service users he came across talked about having recovered. Many felt they were never the same person after their breakdown than they were before. This led him to conclude that recovery was something of a mirage. He offered survival as a better term. Andresen et al (2003), wrote another key paper. They analysed all the service user literature to identify key recovery themes. They felt there were four main components of recovery. These were developing a sense of hope, having a strong personal identity, having some meaning in life and taking personal responsibility for recovery. They also provided a very helpful five stage model of the recovery process, going from a stage they called 'moratorium', where the individual might even be in denial that they have a mental illness, to a final stage of 'growth', where the individual has developed a positive and more meaningful life and is more confident in their ability to manage their illness.

Roberts and Wolfson (2004), provide one of the best descriptions of the recovery approach and contrast it with the traditional medical model. To move forwards towards a recovery focussed service, professionals need to take on more of a coaching role, focus on hope and optimism, negotiate medication issues, work with risk and deliver interventions in a timely manner. Resnick and Rosenheck (2006), were the first authors to draw the connection between positive psychology and recovery. However they note that while positive psychology has followed an academic path and is grounded in scientific research, 'this stands in stark contrast to the recovery movement, a grass roots movement of the disenfranchised that has placed itself apart from the human service professions,' (p.121).

The top 10 recovery policy papers and reports

Of the many policy papers and reports on recovery, we identified 10 key reports, which were NIMHE (2005), Dorrer (2006), Social Perspectives Network (2007), McCormack (2007), Mind (2008), Shepherd et al (2008), Slade (2009,a), Department of Health (2009), Ajayi et al, (2009) and Mental Health Foundation (2009). Of these three stand out. The first is the Social Perspectives Network series of workshops and presentations taken from a study day organised around recovery (Social Perspectives Network, 2007). Amongst other issues, the paper expressed some concerns that recovery would be taken over by professionals and redefined, hence the provocative title, Whose Recovery is it Anyway? In it, Keating expresses the hope that professionals might work in 'meaningful hope inspired relationships' with service users. The Mind Report (2008), also presents the findings from a study day, which generated some quite controversial debate. One commentator challenged the notion of 'employment as the Holy Grail of recovery,' (p.11). The third report has probably been the most influential and it is that produced by the Sainsbury Centre (Shepherd et al, 2008). There are two comments in this report that I feel are especially pertinent to the practice of mental health professionals. The first is the notion of professionals moving from a position of 'being on top to being on tap,' (p.3). The second, is 'a willingness to go the extra mile,' (p.8). In fairness to the authors of this report, both these statements have been taken from other writers, but nonetheless they are interesting for professionals to reflect on.

The top 10 recovery books

In terms of our top 10 books on recovery we cited, Leibrich (1999), Barker et al (1999), Crowley (2000), Repper and Perkins (2003), Roberts et al (2006), Sen (2006), Velleman et al (2007), Davidson et al (2009), Chadwick (2009) and Slade (2009,b). Of these two really stand out for me. The first Leibrich (1999), is to my mind the best book ever written on recovery. It contains 21 accounts of individuals and their battles against mental illness.

It is wonderfully illustrated with photographs and other mementoes from individuals' lives. Julie prefers to use the term 'discovery' rather than recovery. She summarises it thus,

> ... the best way I can describe dealing with mental illness is making our way along an ever widening spiral of discovery in which we uncover problems, discover the best ways to deal with them, recover ground that has been lost, discover new things about ourselves, then uncover deeper problems, discover the best ways....and so on in an intricate process of growth. (Leibrich, 1999, p.181)

An amazing book! The second book that stands out to me is Peter Chadwick's (2009) book, *Schizophrenia: The Positive Perspective.* This is a scholarly account of an individual trying to make sense of his own experience of psychosis, through personal reflection, his amazing knowledge of the research literatures in psychiatry and psychology, and his own personal research work. Some of Peter's insights have been quite remarkable, for example 'The one thing that Laing never really understood, was that madness kills,' (Chadwick, 1995). He has also drawn impressive links between our understanding of psychosis and artistic approaches to psychology, in what is probably my favourite book of his (Chadwick, 2001).

Top 10 recovery websites

In the final section of our review paper, we reported on the top 10 recovery websites. Again to my mind the Recovery Devon website is an amazing resource, with helpful information and resources on a wide range of topics, such as Wellness Recovery Action Planning (WRAP). There is also a video of Dr Glenn Roberts giving a wonderful conference presentation. The Scottish Recovery Network have also been pioneers in British recovery and I cited two reports earlier from their site (Dorrer, 2006; McCormack, 2007). I have also found YouTube to be a fascinating resource. Entering 'recovery from mental illness' into the search bar, brings up hundreds of videos. You can then see legendary figures such as Mary Ellen Copeland, Mary O'Hagan, Priscilla Ridgway, Dan Fisher, Patricia Deegan, all important people in the international recovery movement.

We concluded our selective review by stating that lots of papers, books and reports had appeared in the last few years. This shows how new a lot of the work is and what an exciting time it is to be working in the recovery field. Recovery is about much more than symptomatic improvement. Equally important are social and psychological recovery.

Recovery: Not always welcomed?

The reception of recovery from service users has not always been positive. One commented that I 'had got hooked into the recovery model. P. and I are rather mistrustful of all this especially when his psychologist says it is the big thing in mental health circles these days. Speaking for ourselves we've never seen anyone who has been to the places we have recover. The most people can do is more or less survive at home with the occasional spell as an inpatient.' Another commented, 'As you know I do not believe in, or accept, the concept of the so-called recovery model and wish to have nothing at all to do with it!' You cannot please all of the people all of the time.

Part 3: 'A Bottom-up Approach to Recovery'

In this section I describe a number of small scale local recovery initiatives. I start with the Recovery Group, followed by Recovery Workshops. I then talk about the Recovery Film and the Recovery Journeys booklet. I provide a summary of the series of papers we have written on Recovery Heroes, which feature four of our own local recovery heroes. I describe our Recovery Oscars, a way of recognising the achievements of a number of our service users. Finally, I describe one example of individual recovery based work.

The Recovery Group

Like many things in life, the Recovery Group started serendipitously. When I came to work in Streatham in January 2006, I learned that there was a local Service User Group. After settling into the Teambase, I offered to help Nadir Mothojokan, the nurse who ran these sessions. Even when I tried to inject some extra enthusiasm into these sessions, by arranging extra speakers, it was clear that the User Group was not really developing.

For one session, I had asked a colleague Simon Gent to come along and do a session on music. Even this was only attended by six service users. We reached an all time low when one session was attended by Nadir, a service user and myself. A new approach was needed.

After I had finished a one day workshop on self-esteem (Carson, 2006), I mentioned to the 10 attenders that I was shortly due to be running an event for World Mental Health Day/ Black History Month, at which some of our service users would be exhibiting their art work. One of the participants in the workshop asked me if she could display her own work and also help me organise the event on the day. I gratefully accepted this offer. When I saw the quality of her work, I asked if she might put on an event at the Teambase and give a short talk. This was the first of our Recovery Group sessions. She put together a series of displays which charted the history of her artistic career. The event was attended by around 20 people. Since then, we have had sessions every six to eight weeks. The aims of the group are to allow service users to present their work or ideas to another group of service users, on an issue that is important to them. Second, to try and ensure that these presentations are inspirational. This can involve a lot of work beforehand helping prepare individuals for their sessions. Third, to provide a forum for service users to learn more about recovery, even though they may have left the service. These groups are open to all service users, as well as staff. On average about 15 people attend, of whom 10/11 will be service users and the rest staff. Sarah Morgan and myself have provided a more detailed account of these workshops (Morgan and Carson, 2008).

Following our initial successful first session, Michelle McNary and myself co-presented the second session entitled, 'Recovery from mental illness: do service users hold the keys to our understanding?' This was the first time Michelle had presented her ideas for the Recovery Film in public (of which more in the next section). The third session comprised me interviewing Gordon about his model of recovery. This was attended by over 20 people, including the social worker who had 'sectioned' Gordon under the Mental Health Act, when he had been very unwell. His sister was also present to hear Gordon's presentation and her partner videotaped the session. The fourth session was a presentation from the inspirational Dolly Sen about her own journey of recovery (Sen, 2002; 2006; 2008). This session was only attended by service users, all of whom were able to quiz Dolly about what had helped her and how she coped with suicidal ideation etc. Session five was a combined interview and art exhibition by Ibo, about the role of spirituality and culture in her art. She brought along her drawings, cards and appliqué. The next session was by Margaret Muir on 'Lessons from the university of life.' As the oldest member of the group, Margaret had a lot of wisdom to impart to the rest of us. She divided her life into three sections and told us the story of each stage illustrated by a series of family photographs, music and poetry.

Sarah Morgan presented at our seventh session. She had just completed her masters degree in journalism and indeed had used Ibo's session as a 'colour piece' for her dissertation. In the session she also talked about other pieces of work that she completed, all based around the mental health theme. At the following session I showed the group the Imagine DVD on 'The Secret of Life,' presented by Alan Yentob. (His assistant had sent me a copy of the DVD). I used this to then inform a group discussion along the lines of, 'Self-Help books: self-help or self-harm?' The next session was a presentation entitled 'Can Art Uplift You?' This was a lecture and slide show by Marie-Therese Barrett, a lecturer in art history. This provided a stunning visual display of Eastern and Western Art. The session after was by Matt Ward and was a one man play. The play, 'St. Nicholas,' was written by the Irish playwright, Conor McPherson. This was our longest session as the play lasted one and a half hours. It was followed by a fascinating discussion on the nature of mental illness and whether the play's protagonist was mentally ill. The following session was on 'Poetry for the Soul,' by Liz Mason. Liz brought along and read out a number of poems that had moved and inspired her, and she encouraged others to do the same.

The Recovery Group is a very low cost event to run. It shows how talented the people who use our service actually are. Service users present on topics that they have expertise in. Presentations have all been from local service users with a few exceptions. In June 2009, Peter Chadwick came down from Norwich to do a presentation on positive perspectives on psychosis (Chadwick, 2009). This was attended by 50 people, our largest ever audience at one of these meetings. A second outside presenter was Mark Brown who set up the aspirational lifestyle magazine, 'One in Four.' Towards the end of 2010, we had two inspiring session from Andrew Voyce, who came up from Bexhill and Peter Bullimore, who came down from Sheffield. Another well attended group session was when Rachel Perkins came along to talk about her three psychiatric careers.

The Recovery Group reminds individuals of their own strengths and helps others in the group to reflect on theirs. It fits with the strengths approach now being developed in Positive Psychology (Linley, 2009). How should it be further developed? My own preference would be for the ownership of the group to be taken over by the service users, probably over two stages. First, two service users would be paid a small sum via our Involvement Register

(Reed and Harries, 2008) to co-facilitate the sessions with myself, and to arrange a one-year programme of presentations. A small budget would pay for refreshments as well as a small amount for honoraria. Second, the management and running of the group would be handed over entirely to the service users, assisted by the psychologist, but run independently by them in the community. Fortunately, we received funding from the South London and Maudsley Charitable Trustees to run a one year programme of Recovery Group sessions across the whole Borough. We were therefore able to proceed with stage one in the further development of this initiative.

Recovery workshops

We were very fortunate in Lambeth and Southwark to be provided with four days of recovery training via the Retrain Initiative, developed by Dr Mike Slade and Professor Tom Craig. Thus far, no specific training had been provided for service users. I developed the Recovery Workshops to try and fill this gap. These workshops were run for 10 consecutive afternoons and covered many of the topics that the literature has suggested are important in recovery. The 10 sessions were:

1. Introduction to recovery.
2. Spirituality and hope.
3. Friendship and family.
4. Self-esteem and gratitude.
5. Well-being and lifestyle.
6. Work and leisure.
7. Identity and meaning.
8. Stigma and personal responsibility.
9. Goals and strengths.
10. Reflections and personal journeys.

These afternoon sessions were co-facilitated by myself, an occupational therapist and a service user. For eight of the 10 sessions an outside speaker came along to present on one of the two themes. Half of the outside speakers were also service users. The other presenters have been senior colleagues. Julia Head, the Trust Head of Chaplaincy came along to present on the theme of spirituality in recovery. Sherry Clark talked about well-being and recovery, to mention just two. Group exercises were also used to illustrate specific themes, and readings were provided each week for participants to develop their knowledge of particular topics. The workshops were evaluated using pre and post course evaluations. Thus far, three sets of Recovery Workshops have been run locally, one funded by the Lambeth Executive, the other two by the South London and Maudsley Charitable Trustees.

While this is the first recovery programme for local service users, packages have been developed both in this country and elsewhere. See for example, the Psychosis Revisited pack (Bassett et al, 2003) developed in this country and the Illness Management and Recovery Programme developed by the Substance and Mental Health Services Administration in America (Mueser and Gingerich, 2002; Salyers et al, 2009). While specific protocols are very important for randomised controlled trials and in evidence based practice, I am more concerned with developing programmes that are locally based with local experts and service users and which have as their main goal stimulating participant interest and engagement in the process of recovery. It has proven surprisingly difficult to engage service users from our Recovery and Support Teams in this programme, even though we have provided free workbooks, lunches and handouts, visiting speakers and, an end of course meal in a local restaurant! When I mentioned the level of disability of one of our participants to one of our care co-ordinators, I was told she was the highest functioning person on her caseload!

The Recovery Film and recovery journeys booklet

The Recovery Film was another project that arose serendipitously. Michelle McNary was being seen by my clinical trainees. I decided to take over her psychological therapy personally. I knew that she had a Higher National Diploma in film making as well as a Masters degree. At one of our earlier sessions she told me how she wanted to write a film script, based on her experiences on the Lambeth Early Onset ward, as an inpatient. She was finding it hard to write this script. I suggested she might be having problems with this as she might be too close to the subject matter. Instead I proposed that she might want to make a film about recovery. There were two main obstacles to this idea in my mind. The first, was to do with my own professional credibility. I had never been involved in anything like this before. Was it even part of my job? The second, was the financial aspect. Could we get any monies to make the film? To tackle the first obstacle I approached my long term friend and mentor Dr Frank Holloway. I asked would he be interested in joining a very small project group. He not only agreed to do this, but he also suggested involving Dr Paul Wolfson. Paul was not only another consultant psychiatrist, but a well known recovery expert (Roberts and Wolfson, 2004), who had previously worked in scriptwriting. He also agreed to get involved. To tackle the funding issue, I arranged to meet with Jill Lockett, who was then involved with developing a business strategy within the Trust. I met with Jill and Dan Charlton, the Trust Head of Communications. They had already worked out in advance what they wanted. They wanted a 20 minute film that could be downloaded free from the Internet. Jill set out to try and find the finances. Michelle and I met up with Jill a couple of months later. Michelle had drawn up a budget for £17.5k. Jill suggested that this be extended by an extra £1.5k. We eventually received a budget of £20k to make the film from the Charitable Trustees of the South London and Maudsley NHS Trust. All we had to do now was make the film!

Michelle started recruiting participants for the film. Dr Wolfson and Michelle auditioned people for the film in the summer of 2008 (see McNary, 2008 and Wolfson, 2008, for descriptions of how they did this). Eventually four people were recruited, three from Lambeth and one from Lewisham. Their stories are told in the Recovery Journeys booklet (Carson et al, 2008). The film was completed in May 2010 and can be seen on YouTube, as well as via the Trust website, (www.slam.nhs.uk/patients/recovery.aspx).

To my mind this project will be one of the most important factors in Michelle's own recovery. The film was shortlisted for a Mind Media Award in November 2010, but it lost out to the BBC and Channel 4. My role was to set up the project, to support Michelle along the way, and to make sure the project came to fruition. Now the film is in the public domain, the rest will be up to Michelle. A film about recovery, made by a woman herself in recovery and featuring service users, should be a success. Time will tell.

Recovery Heroes

Recovery Heroes was the title of a series of five papers commissioned by Adam Pozner, the editor of the journal 'A Life in the Day.' I defined recovery heroes as 'individuals whose journey of recovery can inspire both other service users and professionals alike,' (Sen et al, 2009, p.6). Each of the profiles had a similar format. First, we asked the individual who was the subject of the profile, to write a brief personal biography. Second we presented an account of them being interviewed by Sarah Morgan, one of our service users who had just completed her training as a journalist. Third, I gave my personal appraisal of the contributions made by each service user featured.

Dolly Sen was the feature of our first profile (see Chapter 10). She wrote two remarkable accounts of her own traumatic upbringing and her battles with psychosis, (Sen, 2002: Sen, 2006). Dolly first became ill at the age of 14. She then dropped out of school. She identified three things that helped her recover. First, her decision to recover and take personal responsibility. Second, her creativity. Third, a course of cognitive behaviour therapy. In her piece Dolly describes herself as '...a writer, director, artist, filmmaker, poet, performer, raconteur, playwright, mental health consultant, musician and public speaker,' (Sen et al, 2009, p.6). Dolly also presented at one of our Recovery Groups. She advised other service users at this meeting, 'Have big dreams, but take small steps.' A key element of her own personal recovery philosophy has been 'to find the Dollyness of Dolly.' Patricia Deegan expresses a similar sentiment when she reminds us that the goal of recovery, '...is to become the unique, awesome, never to be repeated human being that we are called to be,' (Deegan, 1996).

The second person we featured was Dr Peter Chadwick. I had known Peter since the early 1990s, but it was only in the last few years that we had entered into a regular correspondence. He has written more about his own recovery from psychosis than any other individual (see for instance, Chadwick, 1993; 2001; 2009, and also his two chapters in this volume). To write the feature on him, Sarah and I travelled up to his home in Norwich. Peter has always been concerned to find meaning in his personal experience of psychosis. He summarises this in his own biography thus, '...there is no doubt that my own episode had meaning in terms of my interior life and that examining the realm of meaning was vital, indeed indispensable, to recovery,' (Chadwick et al, 2009, p.7). In her interview with Peter, Sarah drew out the fact that one of Peter's main aims had been to portray the sufferer with psychosis as positively as possible. He reminds us that as well as a search for personal meaning, 'poor accommodation, financial difficulties and no one to properly talk to, are barriers to recovery,' (p.8). Like Patricia Deegan, Peter was writing about the concept of recovery long before it became as important as it is now.

The third person featured in the Recovery Heroes series was Gordon (McManus et al, 2009). Gordon reminds us in his own biography in the paper that he is woken up every day at between 4.00am and 5.00am, by his 'voices' (auditory hallucinations). Consequently he feels he is only halfway to recovery. In her interview, Sarah draws out Gordon's description of what he calls his 'lost years.' He was so ill during these years that he was unable to even fill out a form! The work we have been doing together over the last three years, will hopefully at least partially compensate for this sense of wasted time (see also chapters 1 to 6).

Matt Ward was the fourth person featured in our Recovery Heroes series. He started his own biographical section by stating, 'I am not a recovery hero.' Although relatively recently diagnosed with bipolar disorder, a director saw him give a performance of the play 'St.Nicholas.' On the basis of this, he decided to cast Matt in a play he was directing at the Edinburgh Festival. Matt commented, '... my fellow cast members in the play decided I was the sanest amongst them,' (Ward et al, 2010,a p.7). By the time we wrote the piece with Matt, Sarah Morgan had obtained a job as a journalist, and her place as interviewer was taken on by Hannah Cordle. One of the points that comes across in Hannah's interview with Matt, is that recovery is more about survival. Through his profession as an actor, Matt has brought new insights into our work. He found considerable personal comfort and resonance in the works of Shakespeare. He suggests that Hamlet's 'To be or not to be' soliloquy, is 'probably the best speech ever written with regards to thoughts of suicide,' (p.9). Having started the piece by stating he was not a recovery hero, I ended it by stating that a recovery hero can be seen as someone who is battling against a major mental illness, yet who still manages to inspire others by their deeds and actions. By these criteria, I feel Matt is also a recovery hero.

The fifth and final person in our Recovery Heroes series was Margaret Muir. At a meal to celebrate the completion of a gratitude project, Margaret commented 'We're all heroes!' She explained this further in her biography for the article. 'I believe all who suffer the pain and anguish of mental illness are heroes. Anyone who has survived weeks, months and even years in mental institutions are heroes. Anyone who has spent years dragging themselves out of the abyss is a hero...These people are the unsung heroes,' (Muir et al, 2010). As Margaret also informs us in her biography, she lost her sister when she was only nine years old. This experience with loss as a child led her to conclude later on in life, 'Grief takes as long as it takes.' In her interview with Hannah, Margaret goes on to talk about her gradual involvement with recovery. She co-facilitated the above mentioned gratitude workshops, which helped her realise how much she had to feel thankful for in her own life. Her own definition of recovery is that it is 'peace of mind, hope for the future, thankfulness that I am alive and laughing...'

The concept of Recovery Heroes came from several sources. Patricia Deegan talks about seeing service users as heroes (Deegan, 1996). Premila Trivedi talked about four people being Recovery Heroes, one of whom was

Peter Chadwick. Scott Peck talks about 'the routine heroism of human beings,' (Scott Peck, 1991). On hearing about the concept and having read some of the articles, Julie Leibrich commented, 'And the Recovery Heroes are brilliant! I see them on great black stallions with flowing robes and auras all around,' (Leibrich personal communication). It is not just our service that has Recovery Heroes. Every service has them.

Recovery Oscars

The idea for the Recovery Oscars was a way of acknowledging the unique contributions made by a number of service users over the preceding year and sometimes beyond. While every service user deserves an award, a number of individuals did a bit more and made a difference. For this first set of awards, there were eight categories. The Writing Award went to Gordon. In addition to writing the three chapters of this book in 2009, he was one of the Recovery Heroes (McManus et al, 2009), and he also helped us review the recovery literature (Carson et al, 2010). James Bellamy won the Poetry Award. He was one of the participants in our second set of Recovery Workshops. In these workshops, he composed a poem especially for the session on the meaning of life. He wrote a second poem as a birthday tribute to another course participant. Esther Maxwell-Orumbie received the award for Creative Art. She was the only service user to present her work at all three World Mental Health Day events. She also helped co-facilitate a set of Recovery Workshops and presented at one of the sessions on the theme of personal responsibility. Serena Bentine was given an award for Catering. Serena almost singlehandedly did all the cooking for World Mental Health Day 2009. In addition to preparing all the sandwiches, she also baked cakes, scones and biscuits. Maria Macdonald and her sister Shirley Perrin were given the Double Act of the Year Award. They had presented at our Recovery Group as 'Two Sisters, Two Survivors.' For this they displayed examples of their artwork, as well as giving a talk on how art had impacted on their depressions. Margaret Muir was given the Woman of the Year Award. Margaret has been the 'backbone' of the Recovery Group, has supported every World Mental Health Day event and also helped me facilitate a set of gratitude workshops. Finally, Matt Ward was given the Man of the Year Award. In May, Matt stood in for Dolly at the Lambeth 'Recover Me' conference. He gave the first of several presentations of his story, 'My recovery: a work in progress.' In this, he performs three excerpts from Shakespeare's Macbeth, Hamlet and King Lear, interspersed with his own history with bipolar disorder and his gradual recovery. He also gave a charity performance of the play St.Nicholas in November, which enabled us to pay for our Oscars ceremony. Each award winner received an engraved statuette, a £50 Marks and Spencer's gift voucher and a certificate. The gift vouchers were donated by Conor McGurk, Kim Revell, Max LiPang, Michelle Foster, Ruma Luckeenarain, Jessica Hang Li and Liz Wakely. The presentations took place at the Teambase and several family members were in attendance.

Individual recovery work: Matt Ward's plays

In this section I give an example of a recovery related project that I conducted with a service user.

Shortly after Matt started attending our Recovery Group, he offered to put on a performance of the play 'St. Nicholas.' Perhaps anticipating that this would be something special, I invited Yvonne Farquharson, Performing Arts manager from the Guy's and St. Thomas' Charity to come along and watch the play. On the strength of Matt's performance, Yvonne gave us a small grant with which we put on five performances of the play, at a range of venues in Lambeth. Yvonne wanted us to try and link the play and Matt's personal story into an educational recovery narrative. To do this, I introduced the play, saying something of Matt's background, that he had a bipolar illness and that he was taking medication. After the play, I joined Matt on stage and asked him more about his personal story and how it related to the main protagonist in the play, 'a drunken Irish theatre critic,' who may have had a psychosis. Matt talked about how receiving a diagnosis of bipolar disorder was a great relief to him and about how he had been helped by his contact with local mental health services. We then took questions from the audience. After this, the audience were asked to complete a very short evaluation of the play. They were also given a folder containing Matt's personal story, information about recovery and a copy of the Recovery Journeys book. Evaluations were very positive. Most of the audience found the play to be 'compelling' (mean score = 1.32: maximum possible score was 1 and the lowest score was 5). Most 'admired Matt' more knowing his personal story (mean score = 1.38) and most felt 'theatre was a useful way of learning about mental illness' (mean score = 1.55). Service users in the audience felt that the most helpful aspect of the production was the post play discussion (mean score = 1.31). This suggests that they found learning more about Matt's personal story to be the best element of the production.

My roles in the play were to book all the venues, provide the refreshments at three of the venues and collate all of the handouts and folders. At one stage my whole family was involved in the task of collating the handouts and indeed all four of my adult children attended the last night of the play at St.Thomas' Hospital! The play took over my life in June 2009, yet it also proved to be one of the most inspiring events of my entire professional career. I later co-authored the formal report on the play for the charity and helped write up the first paper for publication (Ward et al, 2010,b). For Matt the main outcome was showing him that despite his recent diagnosis and having to take lithium, he was still able to perform at a very high level, especially given that this is a one man play that lasts 90 minutes.

Part 4:
Assistance on my own journey of recovery

Just as service users are all on their own recovery journeys, so are staff. For me, this has largely been an intellectual journey, which I have then tried to distill into my clinical practice. I mentioned earlier in this chapter and in press how I was initially sceptical about the recovery approach (Carson, 2008). However as I read more about the concept, my approach began to change, and I became more aware of its' positive applications. It is a concept that I have only 'grappled' with seriously since 2006, when the service re-organisation led to me moving from the Norwood Team to the Streatham Team. It is probably fair to say that over the last three to four years, this concept has taken more of my attention than any other, and even now I still feel I only have a developing understanding of the concept. My work has been supported at a number of different levels. These are financial, expert, local collegiate and service user focussed. I will discuss each in turn.

Financial support

In Part 3 of this chapter, I discussed the Recovery Group. Financially this has been incredibly inexpensive. It costs less than £10 to provide the refreshments for the meetings, with additional small increases to purchase some artistic materials for displays. I do all the administrative work for the sessions, including making and distributing the flyers. It is funded through our Community Mental Health Centre budget. Other ventures have required more substantial funding. The most expensive project that I have co-ordinated to date, has been the Recovery Film. This was funded by the Charitable Trustees of the South London and Maudsley NHS Trust. They paid for the cost of making the film, £20k as well as the cost of producing the accompanying Recovery Journeys booklet, an additional £4.7k (Carson et al, 2008). Sandra Lawman the then secretary to the Trustees helped us obtain this funding. In terms of helping individual service users with their own recovery journeys a number of other charities have been very generous. The RL Glasspool Charity and its then Chief Executive Mrs Frances Moore, have made a number of awards to enable the purchase of computing and artistic materials for individual service users. Olivia Wingfield of the Matthew Trust has been very generous and several individuals have benefited from grants from them, as well as the Clapham Relief Fund. The Simon Walker Trust Fund has also made several small awards for the purchase of printers and in one case a digital camera. We collaborated with Yvonne Farquharson of the Guy's and Thomas' Charity on a drama project with Matt Ward, one of our service users, and with Karen Sarkissian from the same charity on a hope and photography project. The Guy's and St.Thomas' Charity also funded the production of 'Psychosis Stories of Recovery and Hope' (Cordle et al, 2011). The Lambeth Executive and the SLaM Charitable Trustees have funded the Recovery Workshops. The SLaM Trustees also paid for a one year programme of Recovery Groups, more Recovery Workshops and a one day service user conference on Recovery, which was held at the Institute of Psychiatry in February 2011. While some of these awards have been quite small financially, they have had a big impact on service users in terms of boosting their hope and showing that others care about their recovery. My cousin Conor McGurk also gave me a significant personal donation that has helped our work, eg. it enabled me amongst other things to buy 50 copies of 'Beyond the Storms,' (Davidson and Lynn, 2009), to give to service users and staff.

Expert support

The advent of the Internet has meant almost instant access to colleagues across the world, time differences notwithstanding, in terms of seeking advice and sharing resources on recovery matters. Dr Julie Leibrich in New Zealand has offered very warm support for our work. Her book remains a major source of inspiration (Leibrich, 1999). Professor Carol Ryff from Wisconsin in the United States has allowed us to use her Well-Being Scales, as well as providing insight into concepts such as 'eudaimonia,' which overlap between positive psychology and recovery. Dr Retta Andresen from Australia has also shared the measures that she and her colleagues have developed, including their innovative work on stages of recovery (Andresen et al, 2003; 2006). Dr Patricia Deegan in the States has also been encouraging, when her busy schedule permits. In this country, Dr Glenn Roberts has been a wonderful source of inspiration and advice. There are countless other professionals and service users who e-mail me regularly with helpful tips and feedback and their own insights into recovery matters, such as Premila Trivedi. Dr Peter Chadwick and myself have been in more regular contact over the last three years, unfashionably by 'snail mail.' Peter has been one of my main personal and intellectual supports. His own work has been hugely influential (Chadwick, 1993; 1995; 2001; 2009).

Local support

Many of the local initiatives that I have developed would not have been possible without the support of many local clinical and managerial colleagues. Within the Streatham CMHT, the team leaders, Charlene DeVilliers, Yasmin Khair, Pamela Patterson, John Hunt and Tolu Mojola have all supported me. Claudette Miller, who has for most of this time been the Recovery and Support Team Leader, has been the most encouraging of new initiatives. Godfried Attafua not only managed the budget for the Recovery Film, but was himself a local pioneer and used to facilitate the User Group, which became the Recovery Group. Godfried has backed every idea that I have ever brought to him. Sam Holmes our centre administrator, Mary O'Connor our receptionist and Myrna Whittle, the Recovery and Support Team administrator, have all been very helpful. Local consultant psychiatrists, Jonathan Beckett, Nicola Byrne, Anne Boocock, Stephen McGowan, Gopal Hegde and Abe Wassie have supported me in working with their patients, and have given helpful feedback that has improved the quality of my recovery work. Dr Indrani Pathmanathan has also helped in the management of a number of people I have worked with. Frank Holloway, has always been a trusted friend and mentor since I first worked with him in 1992, to this day. Within the Lambeth Directorate, Patrick Gillespie, Sonia Burke, Philip Mysliwek, Lesley Bartholomew, Mike Callaghan, Bathma Thailan and Charmaine Leslie have helped with the logistical and financial support needed to run small projects. Adrian Webster and Niesje De Boer, professional heads of clinical psychology and occupational therapy respectively, have been equally encouraging. Professor Tom Craig has been responsible for establishing a number of prestigious projects in Lambeth and is that rare combination of an academic who has 'street cred.' On a wider SLaM perspective, Stuart Bell, Zoe Reed, Dan Charlton, Richard Morley, Russell Guthrie and Jill Lockett have all been very helpful, Jill and Dan especially with the Recovery Film. Tony Coggins and Sherry Clark are helping to develop positive psychology approaches within SLaM and building on well-being initiatives, and have collaborated on a number of projects. Pam Russell has supported the World Mental Health Day/Black History Month events that I have helped co-ordinate in the last few years. Julia Head and Mark Sutherland, both Heads of the Trust Chaplaincy Service, have always been helpful in bringing the spiritual and pastoral dimensions to the recovery work. Ionie Karr, occupational therapist helped co-facilitate one set of local recovery workshops. Sarah Bourne and Nina Whitehouse have been pioneering the vocational approach to recovery in West Norwood and Mark Bertram, similarly in Lambeth. My clinical psychology trainees have also helped out, and I am indebted to Dr Camille Julien, Dr Sally Robinson, Dr Fergus Kane and Cara Kingston. My three honorary assistants Anant Chander, Hannah Cordle and Aisling Treanor have provided more help than anyone. It is sobering to reflect on how many colleagues that have helped me out over the last couple of years. From outside SLaM, these have also included Jean Spencer, Laura Gallagher, Dr Sarah Corlett and Lucy Smith from Lambeth PCT, Pauline Etim-Ubah and Jan Oliver from Fanon and Jonathan Naess from Stand to Reason.

The people I spend most of my life with, are in fact service users. They are my greatest inspiration. Indeed it was working with Gordon that inspired the writing of this book. Until fairly recently I had never written a paper with a service user, with one exception (Stevenson and Carson, 1995), though I had encouraged a couple of service users to share their own stories (Gardiner, 1999; Bellamy, 2000). Over the last six months Sarah Morgan and myself have co-authored a number of papers (Morgan and Carson, 2008; Sen et al,

2009; Chadwick et al, 2009). Michelle McNary has directed and produced the inspiring Recovery Film, Esther Maxwell-Orumbie and Sherrie Dissanayake have co-facilitated recovery workshops and Margaret Muir has helped with a number of presentations and gratitude workshops. Liz Wakely and myself developed a second series of heroes papers, but this time on historical recovery heroes. We have published a number of papers on Churchill (Wakely and Carson, 2010), Florence Nightingale (Wakely and Carson, 2011,a), Charles Darwin (2011,b), with a fourth on Isaac Newton (Wakely and Carson, 2011,c). We wrote a book chapter on Abraham Lincoln (Wakely and Carson, 2011,d) and indeed have added an extra 10 contemporary recovery heroes for our new book, 'Mental Health Recovery Heroes Past and Present,' (Davies et al, 2011). Our service users are both our greatest teachers and our best source of inspiration and as I never tire of reminding people, for the second time in this chapter, 'Whose Recovery Is It Anyway?' It is of course the service users' (Social Perspectives Network, 2007).

Conclusions

I started this chapter by providing a summary of my professional career and my own personal journey of recovery. My own journey reflects the wider journey that psychiatry has made from asylum based care to community care. My conversion to the recovery cause has been a comparatively recent one, although I was privileged to hear Patricia Deegan talk about 'recovery as a journey of the heart,' as far back as 1996 in Rotterdam, Holland (Deegan, 1996). I then summarised the literature on recovery. The definition of recovery given by the American psychologist Bill Anthony, is amongst the most cited. Paradoxically the definition offered by Gordon is not just more succinct, but may be more useful clinically (McManus, 2008; McManus et al, 2009). Gordon suggested that 'recovery is coping with your illness and having a meaningful life.' At a recent presentation a service user exclaimed, 'I haven't had any meaning in my life for eight years!' The challenge for all of us as recovery workers, is to help individuals cope with their mental illnesses, and as far as possible, to also help them to lead a life that is more meaningful to them. Hopefully a lot of the recovery work that I described in Part 3 does this. For Michelle, I hope that making the Recovery Film will lead her to her having a tremendous sense of achievement and recognition, wherever the film is shown. For Matt, I hope that his involvement with our services has shown how much he can give back to others less fortunate than himself, as he so often acknowledges. For Gordon, I hope this book lets him see that he can be a revolutionary after all, though in the field of mental health and not communist politics, where he thought he would make his enduring contribution to life. For all the service users involved with our recovery services, that your life is enriched through your contact with us. While Rachel Perkins has talked about professionals being 'on tap not on top,' for me this means working much more in partnerships, in which each of us has a particular and unique role to play. Finally, I described the huge amount of support that I have received with this work from local, national and international sources. Recovery from severe mental illness may be about lots of individual stories and journeys of personal recovery, but lots of other people need to become involved along the way if services are to be truly recovery focussed.

References

Ajayi, S. Billsborough, J. Bowyer, T. Brown, P. Hicks, A. Larsen, J. Mailey, P. Sayers, R. and Smith, R. (2009) *Getting back into the World: Reflections of Lived Experience of Recovery*. Rethink Recovery Series. Volume 2. London: Rethink.

Andresen, R. Oades, L. and Caputi, P. (2003). The experience of recovery from schizophrenia: towards an empirically validated stage model. *Australian and New Zealand Journal of Psychiatry*, 37, 5, 586-594.

Andresen, R. Caputi, P. and Oades, L. (2006) Stages of Recovery Instrument: development of a measure of recovery from severe mental illness. *Australian and New Zealand Journal of Psychiatry*, 40, 10, 972-980.

Anthony, W (1993) Recovery from mental illness: guiding vision of mental health service systems in 1990s. *Psychosocial Rehabilitation Journal*, 16, 4, 11-23.

Barker, P. Campbell, P. and Davidson, B. (Eds) (1999) *From the Ashes of Experience: Reflections on Madness, Survival and Growth*. London: Whurr.

Bassett, T. Cooke, A. and Read, J. (2003) *Psychosis Revisited: A workshop for mental health workers*. Brighton: OLM-Pavilion.

Bellamy, J. (2000) Can you hear me thinking? *Psychiatric Rehabilitation Journal*, 24, 1, 73-75.

Carson, J. (2006) *Be Your Own Self-Esteem Coach*. London: Whiting and Birch.

Carson, J. Holloway, F. Wolfson, P. and McNary, M. (Eds) (2008) *Recovery Journeys: Stories of coping with mental health problems*. London: South London and Maudsley NHS Foundation Trust.

Carson, J. (2008) Recovery: where now? In, Carson, J. et al (Eds) op cit.

Carson, J. McManus, G. and Chander, A. (2010) Recovery: a selective review of the literature and resources. *Mental Health and Social Inclusion*, 14, 1, 35-44.

Chadwick, P. (1993) The stepladder to the impossible: a firsthand phenomenological account of a schizoaffective psychotic crisis. *Journal of Mental Health*, 2, 239-250.

Chadwick, P. (1995) *Understanding Paranoia: what causes it, how it feels and what to do about it?* London: Thorsons.

Chadwick, P. (2001) *Personality as Art: Artistic Approaches in Psychology*. Ross-on-Wye: PCCS Books.

Chadwick, P. (2006) Peer-professional first-person account: schizophrenia from the inside- phenomenology and the integration as causes and meanings. *Schizophrenia Bulletin*, 33, 1, 166-173.

Chadwick, P. (2009) *Schizophrenia: The Positive Perspective. Explorations at the outer reaches of human experience*. London: Routledge.

Cordle, H. Fradgley, J. Carson, J. Holloway, F. & Richards, P. (2011) *Psychosis Stories of Recovery and Hope*. London: Quay Books.

Crowley, K. (2000) *The Power of Procovery in Healing Mental Illness*. Los Angeles: Kennedy Carlisle Publishing.

Davidson, L. and Lynn, L. (Eds) (2009) *Beyond the Storms: Reflections on personal recovery in Devon*. Exeter: Devon Partnership NHS Trust.

Davidson, L. Lawless, M. and Leary, F. (2005) Concepts of recovery: competing or complimentary? *Current Opinion in Psychiatry*, 18, 6, 664-667.

Davidson, L. Tondora, J. Lawless, M. O'Connell, M. and Rowe, M. (2009) *A Practical Guide to Recovery-Oriented Practice*. Oxford: Oxford University Press.

Davies, S. Wakely, E. Morgan, S. & Carson, J. (2011) *Mental Health Recovery Heroes Past and Present*. Brighton: OLM-Pavilion.

Deegan, P. (1988) Recovery: the lived experience of rehabilitation. *Psychosocial Rehabilitation Journal*, 11, 4, 11-19.

Deegan, P. (1996) Recovery as a journey of the heart. *Psychiatric Rehabilitation Journal*, 19, 3, 91-97.

Department of Health (2009) *New Horizons: Towards a Shared Vision for Mental Health*. London: Department of Health.

Dorrer, N. (2006) *Evidence of Recovery: the ups and downs of longitudinal outcome research*. Glasgow: Scottish Recovery Network.

Gardiner, E. (1999) Raising the Titanic. *Openmind*, 99, 20-21.

Jacobson, N. and Greenley, D. (1991) What is recovery: a conceptual model and explication. *Psychiatric Services*, 52, 4, 482-485.

Kruger, A. (2000) Schizophrenia: Recovery and hope. *Psychiatric Rehabilitation Journal*, 24, 1, 29-37.

Leff, J. (Ed) (1997) *Care in the Community: Illusion or Reality?* Chichester: Wiley.

Leibrich, J. (1999) *A Gift of Stories*. Dunedin: University of Otago Press.

Liberman, R. and Kopelowicz, A. (2005) Recovery from schizophrenia: a concept in search of research. *Psychiatric Services*, 56, 6, 735-742.

Linley, A. (2008) *Average to A+: Realising Strengths in Yourself and Others*. Warwick: Centre for Applied Positive Psychology Press.

McCormack, J. (2007) *Recovery and Strengths Based Practice*. Glasgow: Scottish Recovery Network.

McManus, G. (2008) Gordon's story. In, Carson, J. et al (Eds) op cit.

McManus, G. Morgan, S. Fradgley, J. and Carson, J. (2009) Recovery heroes- a profile of Gordon McManus. *A Life in the Day*, 13, 4, 16-19.

McNary, M. (2008). Making the Recovery Film: Michelle's story. In Carson, J. et al (Eds) op cit.

Mental Health Foundation (2009) *Recovery in Action Project Report*. London: Mental Health Foundation.

Mind (2008) *Life and Times of a Supermodel: The recovery paradigm for mental health*. MindThink Report 3. London: Mind.

Morgan, S. and Carson, J. (2008) The recovery group: a service user and professional perspective. *Groupwork*, 19, 1, 26-39.

Mueser, K. and Gingerich, S. (Eds) (2002) *Illness Management and Recovery Implementation Kit*. Rockville, Maryland: Substance Abuse and Mental Health Services Administration.

Muir, M. Cordle, H. and Carson, J. (2010) Recovery heroes- a profile of Margaret Muir. *Mental Health and Social Inclusion*, 14, 2, 7-11.

National Institute for Mental Health in England (2005) *NIMHE Guiding Statement on Recovery*. London: Department of Health.

Onken, S. Craig, C. Ridgway, P. Ralph, R. and Cook, J. (2007) An analysis of the definitions and elements of recovery: a review of the literature. *Psychiatric Rehabilitation Journal*, 31, 1, 9-22.

Reed, Z. and Harries, B. (2008) Co-production, time banks and mental health. *A Life in the Day*, 12, 1, 8-11.

Repper, J. and Perkins, R. (2003) *Social Inclusion and Recovery: A model for mental health practice*. London: Balliere Tindall.

Resnick, S. and Rosenheck, R. (2006) Recovery and Positive Psychology: parallel themes and potential synergies. *Psychiatric Services*, 57, 1, 120-123.

Roberts, G. and Wolfson, P. (2004) The rediscovery of recovery: open to all. *Advances in Psychiatric Treatment*, 10, 1, 37-48.

Roberts, G. Davenport, S. Holloway, F. and Tattan, T. (2006) *Enabling Recovery: Principles and Practice of Rehabilitation Psychiatry*. London: Gaskell.

Salyers, M. Godfrey, J. McGuire, A. Gearhart, T. Rollins, A. and Boyle, C. (2009) Implementing the Illness Management and Recovery Program for consumers with severe mental illness. *Psychiatric Services*, 60, 4, 483-490.

Scott Peck, M. (1991). Foreword. In, Catford, L. and Ray, M. *The Path of the Everyday Hero*. New York: Jeremy P. Tarcher/Putnam.

Sen, D. (2002) *The World is Full of Laughter*. Brentwood: Chipmunka Publishing.

Sen, D. (2006) *Am I Still laughing?* Brentwood: Chipmunka Publishing.

Sen, D. (2008) Dolly's story. In Carson, J. et al (Eds) *Recovery Journeys: Stories of coping with mental health problems*. London: South London and Maudsley NHS Foundation Trust.

Sen, D. Morgan, S. and Carson, J. (2009) Recovery heroes- a profile of Dolly Sen. *A Life in the Day*, 13, 2, 6-8.

Shepherd, G. Boardman, J. and Slade, M. (2008) *Making Recovery a Reality*. London: Sainsbury Centre for Mental Health.

Slade, M. (2009,a) *100 Ways to Support Recovery: A guide for mental health professionals*. Rethink Recovery Series: Volume 1. London: Rethink.

Slade, M. (2009,b) *Personal Recovery and Mental Illness: A Guide for Mental Health Professionals*. Cambridge: Cambridge University Press.

Social Perspectives Network (2007) *Whose Recovery is it Anyway?* London: Social Perspectives Network.

Stevenson, V. and Carson, J. (1995) The pastoral myth of the mental hospital: a personal account. *International Journal of Social Psychiatry*, 41, 2, 147-151.

Velleman, R. Davis, E. Smith, G. and Drage, M. (Eds) (2007) *Changing Outcomes in Psychosis: Collaborative Cases from Practitioners, Users and Carers*. Oxford: BPS Blackwell.

Wakely, E. & Carson, J. (2010) Historical recovery heroes- Winston Churchill. *Mental Health and Social Inclusion*, 14, 4, 36-39.

Wakely, E. & Carson, J. (2011,a) Historical recovery heroes- Florence Nightingale. *Mental Health and Social Inclusion*, 15, 1, 24-28.

Wakely, E. & Carson, J. (2011,b) Historical recovery heroes- Charles Darwin. *Mental Health and Social Inclusion*, 15, 2, 66-71.

Wakely, E. & Carson, J. (2011,c) Historical recovery heroes- Isaac Newton. *Mental Health and Social Inclusion*, 15, 3, 122-128.

Wakely, E. & Carson, J. (2011,d) Abraham Lincoln. In, Davies et al (Eds) *Mental Health Recovery Heroes*. Brighton: OLM-Pavilion.

Ward, M. Cordle, H. Fradgley, H. and Carson, J. (2010,a) Recovery heroes- a profile of Matthew Ward. *Mental Health and Social Inclusion*, 14, 1, 6-10.

Ward, M. Chander, A. Robinson, S. Farquharson, Y. and Carson, J. (2010,b) It's a one man show. *Mental Health Today*, March, 32-33.

Warner, R. (2009) Recovery from schizophrenia and the medical model. *Current Opinion in Psychiatry*, 22, 4, 374-380.

Whitwell, D. (1999) The myth of recovery from mental illness. *Psychiatric Bulletin*, 23, 10, 621-622.

Wolfson, P. (2008) Auditioning for recovery. In Carson, J. et al (Eds) op cit.

8

From teddy boy to teddy bear, from barbells to bar-belle: On growth via psychosis, sin and love

Peter Chadwick

Peter describes his childhood persona as '...a little buttercup of a boy like me was a delicate efflorescence trying to grow in the burning fires of Hell.' It was certainly tough for him 'up North.' His journey from insanity to recovery was a journey to become who he truly was. His luck he feels changed, from dealing with so-called 'mind wrecking' people before his psychotic breakdown aged 33, to 'mind healing' people after it, especially his very accepting wife Jill. In the chapter Peter also shares many of his tips for recovery. He argues that it was important for him to focus on meaningfulness and self-realisation, rather than competitiveness. He also suggests that as a professional writer, he almost wrote himself well. Perhaps controversially, he challenges the notion of being proud to be mad. 'If you're proud to be mad you'll never have the motivation to get out of it.' He argues that sufferers need to think what their 'marvellous manic madness' may be doing to their family and friends. Recovery he argues, is something that people need to actively work at. He comments, '...live via meaning...give oneself over to something more important than oneself....'

Sometimes a False Self can be a Caretaker Self, protecting the Real Self until it is safe for it to emerge. Donald Winnicott (Psychoanalyst).

How can you genuinely grow, as a person, in a society where everything is a dimension of competition? Human beings are not giant cucumbers at a show. Peter Chadwick.

I am a decadent man, I am an anarchistic man..... there is something wrong with my kidneys. Were Dostoyevsky to read this from The Beyond, he might say 'Ah! This is my Underground Man risen in the 21st Century!' And he would be right. I have a lived a nomadic life, I have lived a subversive life, I have lived a dangerous life.

In explaining this a little further, the reader may think, 'Well this isn't of much relevance to me, I'm not like that'. But really the example I make of myself has quite a wide relevance. This is because it shows how you can be induced to madness by being a member of an abused, stigmatised minority group but also the ways in which you can put it all behind you and move on.

There are many things in life from which it may take a person many years, even decades, to recover. For example, you can have psychoanalysis five times a week for three years; you can be brought up by nuns in a convent school; you can do a degree in philosophy at Oxford or you can be a bisexual transvestite and be brought up in the north of England just after the war against Hitler. The reader can probably guess which was me.

Despite my knowledge of biology, cognition, psychoanalysis and so on, it often crosses my mind that my illness, really, was 'all politics'. Sexual politics, gender politics or some such thing. In a country where masculinity was radicalised, or rather, continued to be radicalised by two world wars and heavy industry, a little buttercup of a boy like me was like a delicate efflorescence trying to grow in the burning coals of Hell. As Dylan Thomas would understand, my mother had 'laid an egg by tigers'. No wonder my personality by 1966, when I was 20, was distorted and indeed perverted out of all recognition. What on earth was I *doing* being, as I was, a Lancashire weightlifting champion and (a bit later) a trainee boxer?! It was ludicrous!

When asking of myself, 'How *really* did my recovery from insanity take place?' the answer is not complicated, it's quite simple: It was a journey to become who I really am – and to be who I really am without shame and without apologies, regret or remorse. It was a matter of becoming my Real Self, yet with peace and quiet in my head.

Now 65, ironically bisexual transvestism as an orientation has left me, all that was out of my system about two decades ago, though the tendencies had massively weakened by the age of 34. As a happily married man it is possible to say inwardly to myself while going about daily life, 'This is me, this is who I really am' – *and* feel perfectly OK about it. That is what you have to aim for. 'Know thyself, be thyself', as Oscar Wilde knew in the end, is not a life of relentless rebellion but a life of peace.

This chapter started with striking claims. My life has indeed been like that and I take full responsibility for it. My past is part of me, it is all coded away there in the neural networks of my brain. There is no wish within to disown it.

Dangerous decadence

Transvestites are naturally – to a greater or lesser extent – rather feminine men, we don't really *like* the macho style of western masculinity, though we may role-play it, which is why we need periodically to have a mental holiday away from it. In the Orient, cross-gender males are much more accepted because they symbolise the integration of Yin and Yang. There is no such attitude, to any really serious degree, in the relatively one-eyed West.

The first 20 years of my life was like a training for the army. It was the psychological hangover effect of the war. Even my hard-faced mother contributed to it: 'You've gotta be as hard as *nails* in this wuuurld!' she would say with a snarling expression on her face. In Manchester in those days (though not so much now) nothing was lower and more despicable than 'a poof'.

Transvestism has a lot more to do with a young boy's relationship with his father or father substitutes than any 'mother fixation'. After my father's early death in 1954, the males I grew up among in the north, in the 1950s and early 1960s, were not my kind of people at all. They were violent, cruel, sly, snide, disloyal, foul-mouthed, totally cynical, arrogant, 'piss-taking' and looked down on women from a self-styled great height. Why should I want to be a man? The Model of Man given to me was ugly, cruel and basically revolting. It didn't 'mirror' anything within at all – so I had to act all the time, I felt like an empty shell, psychologically *starved*.

Freud recognised that sometimes a person's sexuality can exist like a protected psychic capsule there in their mind, discordant with, and as if protected from, the rest of their mental processes. It was rather like that for me. It was a terrible conflict to have a kind of army-style upbringing and yet at the same time be fighting to keep the feminine, that was longing for expression and validation, down and in.

My psychotic episode in 1979, at 33, was psychologically quite straightforward and even rather predictable. When 20 I had decided that my silly macho mask was all too simplistic. There was a lot more to me than that, as girlfriends, if not my mother, had noticed. Over the years it gradually dropped away and in 1974, when 27, it seemed time to stop fighting against transvestism and indulge it. Needless to say, things still being as they were in this country in those days, I was overheard in my dreadfully poorly soundproofed flat and outed Big Time – ironically by a broken nosed macho man. How symbolic. With a mind trained, especially at school, to think of men as vicious homophobic, transvestophobic slanderers, I became increasingly paranoid over the next five years until breaking down with horrific, sadistic, persecutory delusions in the summer of 1979. It was how my mind had been trained to think people, at least men and hard-faced women, would behave towards a 'sissy boy' like me. It was simply a matter of fearing the worst. It was what I was used to. My delusions were existentially true, my upbringing had taught me to think – particularly via the Nazi-style bullies in the school's Upper Sixth – that people *really would* go to all that trouble and behave in that murderous persecutory way towards a 'pansy'. After all, in 1977-79 I was even going out on the town, in drag with men, as a delightful blonde in stilettos (a bar-belle). At least I was really good at what I was doing.

But, really, in a world where feminine men were accepted as just part of the normal fabric of life, the breakdown would *never* have occurred. It is true, in a way it *was* 'all sex and gender politics'. The Sex and Gender Fascists had been signalling: 'If you're not like us we will destroy you!' The Stasi and the Gestapo would have approved. With a rearing like mine, and also with a Chadwick family-hating mother who held me in contempt for what I really was as a person, perhaps many people would have gone paranoidly psychotic if they'd have been in the same situation as me. All you needed was this abusive upbringing, among The Masculinity and Heterosexuality Thought Police, which left you feeling that you hardly had the right to exist at all on this planet, plus a rather overactive imagination. Betrayal and unfortunate coincidences would do the rest. Before long you're thinking, 'They're out to kill me!' After all 'We didn't beat Hitler with poofs like him!'

Getting a life

Different perspectives on the fine details of this psychotic episode have been written on a number of previous occasions (Chadwick, 1992; 1993; 2001a, b; 2003; 2008). I won't repeat them here. Fortunately my recovery from it was pretty well complete, as a problem it was solved and I have had no further periods of illness or crisis ('relapses') since. Indeed I have felt a lot better since the episode than I was before. In a way a real corner in my life was turned. So, how does one recover from a predicament of that kind?

The psychosis itself, I have to admit, seemed to 'boil' something – perhaps a trace of mania – out of my being. But really my recovery was very much about genuine love and acceptance (something I had never known before the episode) leading to growth. In that respect it was also like a way of thinking pioneered by Carl Rogers (1961, 1980) and so, in a sense, is always ongoing, right to death.

Living as eventually I did in West London, just along from Earls Court, a very liberal area of Europe, gave me a situation where there was no need to worry any more about hostile, right wing attitudes to my sexuality. West London in the 1980s was not Manchester in the 1950s and early 1960s. Totally accepting neighbours and transvestite and transsexual friends greatly strengthened me and I met and married a woman who thought transvestism was 'just a laugh'. She didn't see it as portentous or threatening at all – whereas some previous girlfriends, before the episode, had thought my activities were, as one put it, 'vile and despicable'.

In a way my luck changed, from interfacing with 'mind-wrecking' people before the psychosis to 'mind-healing' people after it. Post-episode, macho men and hard-headed women were definitely OFF my list of contacts. In London it *was* possible to live like that, in the way I preferred. London people gave me back my mind and indeed healed my soul. I owe everything to them. It is heartbreaking for me now to see the city wracked by knife crime.

My off-centre sexual behaviour dropped away as there was plenty of opportunity to express my femininity in the teaching, research and writing that I did. There was no need any more to 'dress' to express it. My educational background in very materialistic, reductionist, 'tough minded' science I also jettisoned as I taught, researched and wrote increasingly on qualitative methods and on artistic and spiritual matters (e.g. Chadwick, 1995a, b; 2001b, c; 2006a; 2007a). The orthodoxy of course looked on with its usual cynical eye.

My true way has been that of 'people, words, feelings and expression', the female way, not 'weapons, machines, getting rich, reason and fact', the male way. Commensurate with this, I have no great interest in seeing people as machines – knowledge-seeking (*scientia*) doesn't *have* to be obsessed with the masculine 'Machine Metaphor' of person. But if you're brought up to hold in contempt, and be ashamed of, what you are, it is a life process to get out of that 'story' or thumbnail sketch about yourself. You don't do it in eight sessions of CBT. It takes a lot of time and you have to reconstruct a personal narrative via life, not only – and sometimes (let's face it) not at all – in the consulting room.

The only things that were not changed by me after the 1979 debacle were my sex and my bank. I changed my circle of friends, where I lived, the kind of work I did, my girlfriend, my attitude to my work and indeed the very metaphors, like 'Hard man' and 'truth warrior' on which I'd built so much of my previous style of life. 'Man as flower' and 'Shaman' were now far more useful and appropriate.

Meeting so many more peaceful, kind and gentle *men* in the southeast of England also gradually changed my inner model of what a man is. It no longer felt tense and uncomfortable in the male role and male identity. That also defused the need for transvestism, because there was no longer any 'vile male identity' from which to get away. Being a man became a good thing not a cruel, nasty thing.

The nitty-gritty of recovery

On a more workaday note, getting back into employment and thus having a job (J), finding adequate accommodation (A) and having money from a half-decent income (M) also were important in the early days of recovery. Having 'JAM' gave me the more secure foundations on which to rebuild my life.

Meeting and loving my wife Jill, who actually first encountered me in the day hospital at Charing Cross while I was still an in-patient, and getting on to a tiny dose of haloperidol medication that was really suitable, all these things were helpful. Indeed the medication didn't turn me into someone I wasn't. It instead helped to remove the barriers that were preventing me from being who I am. Well targeted medication often does do that.

An important therapeutic aspect of my relationship with Jill is that she is not a 'high EE' (Expressed Emotion) partner. Though we have our usual bickering, she is not (as my mother was) over-involved and over-protective or, for that matter, guilt-inducing and over-talkative, all processes that tend to weaken the stability of the psyche (see Bebbington and McGuffin, 1988). When critical, Jill also tends to attack my behaviour rather than my character *viz*: 'That was a daft thing to do!' rather than (what I had from my mother as a child): 'Yer bloody swine!'

With Jill and my close friends I've always been able to talk about anything and everything, however embarrassing, so nothing festers away because of being bottled up. All of this kind of thing is important in helping one to be accepting of both positive and negative experiences in life. It means one doesn't have to use the childish defence of denial all the time to get through. Because we love each other unconditionally we also accept one another for who we are.

My horrific experiences at the hands of the homophobic bullying ring at school (almost all football people) I've managed to turn round into something productive in the short story writing I do. For example I've had them as concentration camp guards (they'd have loved it) and Gestapo-style interviewers in a world where Hitler won the war (e.g. Chadwick, 2006b); I've had one of them having anal intercourse with Oscar Wilde's lover Bosie Douglas and generally utilised them as shady characters in stories aimed to be psychologically enlightening. It is always contaminating to interface with audience-needing Nazis, which basically is what they were (like eating 'off' food), but the trick is to utilise the experience creatively not ruminatively.

Generally my dealings with the professionals in charge of my 'case' have been productive. I was willing to listen and learn from them and I think my decision to stay on medication, as they advised, has been to my benefit, though I take as little as possible so as to minimise the threat of tardive dyskinesia, a movement disorder that can be associated with long term (and indeed occasionally even short term) use of anti-psychotics. I use a variable dose regime, depending on psychological circumstances, not a fixed dose regime and have taken very few drug holidays – perhaps only half a dozen in the last 30 years. Because of being allowed by my G.P.s to be on a variable dose I can always reduce dosage if sluggishness becomes a problem. It was extremely helpful to have had over the years, G.P.s who didn't overreact if I became somewhat fragile. They said that these little 'blips' were to be expected, there was no question of them recommending me for readmission at the slightest sign of difficulties. This, in itself, enabled *me* not to overreact when bad times were upon me and so helped me to get through and accept ups and downs as just inevitable aspects of life.

With reference to cognitions, it was very important to learn from research on psychological processes, including my own (e.g. Chadwick, 1992, 1997b). I became extremely wary of confirmation bias (Wason, 1960), the bias only to seek data and ideas that confirm one's thoughts and beliefs and this helped me to avoid jumping to conclusions, the JTC bias (Garety and Freeman, 1999) and to avoid the bias to overly spectacular interpretations of events. One also has to be wary of over-processing what are really just coincidences in a terribly meaningful and portentous way and also to recognise that trust is an act of courage.

Being mindful of my own strengths and capacities as areas of my psychological life that I could develop also was important and an important counterweight to all the research on deficits and dysfunctions that one finds in the psychological and psychiatric literature.

In the early days of recovery however I have to admit that it was vital to re-learn how to do simple things like go into a shop and buy a newspaper without getting paranoid thoughts about the people in there. Doing such things with friends ('peer support') from the psychiatric aftercare hostel where I lived for a time was particularly helpful as I knew that they had been through what I'd been through. Certainly in the early post-recovery period, these basic practical things are far more important than deep, and potentially very disturbing, soul-searching. Things like that can come later when one is stronger and able to withstand more emotional buffeting.

I was very fortunate in being able to get back into full-time work *gradually* by taking on more and more part-time teaching with The Open University, Birkbeck College, The City Literary Institute and various other faculties. By 1992-3, 13 years after the crisis, I was teaching no less than 16 different courses a year and working 60-100 hours a week! Because I love the subject and the students I could indeed do this but in the long term there have been costs in terms of damage to my physical health (see later).

It was best to avoid cocaine, ecstasy, cannabis, opiates, LSD, amphetamine and large quantities of alcohol ('overdrinking') like the plague. I tried also to maintain a high level of sensitivity to the events of my own private mental life so as to be watchful of even the *slightest* tendency to relapse. Competitiveness did not seem to bring the best out of me so I focussed my life on meaningfulness and self realisation, not at all on 'winning', 'coming top' or 'feeling good'. As a professional writer as well as psychologist, to some extent I also wrote myself well again.

It was better to have a positive attitude to myself but, having said this, it is one thing to be proud of the genuine capacities that psychosis-prone people have, such as creativity, sensitivity generally, spiritual sensitivity, empathy and depth of feeling. But it is quite another to be proud to be actually mad. If you're proud to be mad you'll never have the motivation to get out of it. At times like that, people need to think of their family, friends, partner, children and neighbours. They need to think of what their 'marvellous manic madness' is doing to *them*. It is no voluptuous glow in the head for them.

Spirituality

The products of academic psychology were sadly pretty useless in dealing with the very important issue in my life of my relationship with God. This is the problem of having a subject based on an ideology of scientific humanism and simply that which can be physically observed. 'Psychology' collapses into 'brain and behavioural science', basically anthroponomy and not psychology at all. Virtually all the psychologists I had read and spoken with about the spiritual were materialistic atheists. They seemed to behave as if they were signalling, 'There's no God, no soul, no afterlife, no angels, no meaning, no purpose, not even any *mind*, just brain..... but we're so tough we can live with this..... now toughen up and join us'. To which, as a Pantheist, my reaction was one of barely contained despair at the utter skin-deep 'intellectual machismo' and superficial crassness of it all. I was *back* with the ambience of the 1950s and early 1960s! Those half-witted macho people were everywhere! ('No sloppy, soft underbelly thinking for us!').

Fortunately many talks with vicars about my distorted, savage view of God, that was 'on sale' in earlier decades, were extremely helpful. Their words helped me to see Him as more loving, compassionate and understanding.

Though God is a God of love and compassion, nonetheless my hatred for my abusers and for people like them has been, not a hindrance, but a powerful, growth promoting force in helping me to get away from everything they stood for and to elaborate my own identity and style of life. Centrally one grows through love and *unconditional* acceptance. In that respect the love of my wife, close friends and students over the decades has been vital. But hatred also has its value in defining, and helping one to revolt against, all that one does NOT want to be. As Freud knew, it always is useful to have enemies.

The voice within

In the end, in this business of recovery, knowing a lot of facts and having a lot of money, fame, celebrity, none of those things, all so valued, of course, in this country, are of much significance or help. You have to listen to the sometimes drowned-out voice within. You have to be true to your capacities and talents, not your ambitions, be guided by vitality and passion and march to your own distant drummer – not the drum of the orthodoxy. Recovery is YOUR recovery, it is not anybody else's and your actions are YOUR actions, not anybody else's. When push comes to shove, your life and how you live it is your choice. But you don't *have* to live by just doing the done thing – the Nazis, after all, were very good at that.

When I was in my early twenties, I asked my mother why she hadn't accepted me for what I was and tried to encourage my more tender qualities like protectiveness feelings, sensitivity, compassion and the like. She stood there with her head slightly down, saucer but sad eyed, and said forlornly,

'Oh..... I tried to knock all that out of yer'. The reader can see, I hope, from all this that 'going mad' is something that happens to a person *as* a person – to the totality of what they are. It is not just a feature of an overactive electrochemical brain pathway or a serious cerebral hemisphere imbalance, even if things like that are involved (*viz*: 'illness'). To understand it and help people recover to satisfying, meaningful and fulfilling lives (not just remove symptoms) one needs a 'Total Psychology' attitude – respecting the entirety that is person. Thus one needs to recognise the importance of everything from biology to politics and spirituality. Knowledge is a unity, boundaries between subjects, and territoriality, in principle, are irrelevant *and* harmful. Just 'silly power games'.

In a way my decadent, nomadic life has promoted, at least mentally and spiritually, not decay and degeneration but growth. Few but Oscar Wilde would really understand this. My pen has created a lot in praise of the feminine in men, both above ground (e.g. Chadwick, 2001c; 2007b) and in underground periodicals (e.g. Chadwick, 1979a, 1997a). Some of these radical sex and gender pieces, praising the Dionysian way, are highly threatening to men of war, the building site and the football terraces and I have, as a subversive, had to pay the price of the expected invasions of my privacy. This is not a very free country.

But my adoration of the feminine was something to go *into*, not fight against, or my life would not have been a life at all, only an existence. Fritz Perls, the founder of Gestalt Therapy, would understand this, he often used to say 'Don't *resist* the compulsion, do it *more!*' Transvestism is not a perversion, it's a message, a little voice from the depths to the surface about who you are but wrapped in sexy packaging so as to help it get through.

Reflections

Recovery, to me, and to all the people I've known who are now fully well, is something actively to work at. It is not something to leave to the doctors or leave to the pills to do the trick. The aim also should be positive, not just 'staying out of hospital'. The important thing is to live via *meaning*, not just to feel good or be happy, but to give oneself over to something more important than oneself, whatever it is – and to realise capacities and talents rather than just correct biases and deficits.

The literature of the human sciences is replete with behavioural evidence and findings about dysfunction and disorder. 'A vocabulary of denigration'

R.D. Laing called it (1960) and a 'discourse of deficit' in the words of Ken Gergen (1990). But in the business of recovery the subjective voice is that which must be heard and a focus on positive potentials and aspirations vital. This is something that most, if not all, behavioural scientists just cannot and will not comprehend.

It is worth saying however that people can be too focussed just on recovery. Most sufferers also want to know what *caused* their episode and how their crisis was brought about. If one knows what the antecedent factors were, one can start to make things so that the slide into psychosis doesn't happen again. If one is blind to what actually led to 'the experience of overwhelm', or whatever one chooses to call it, it never will be really clear what to change and avoid so as to prevent it happening again.

Psychosis sufferers often are highly sensitive people. To turn sensitivity around and make of it an asset rather than a liability, it is necessary to avoid coarse, boorish, blunt people and mix with persons who will 'mirror' what is within. Writers and poets tend to do this to a degree lacking in the average person. In the business of recovery, behavioural science does not by any means have all the answers as, in its thirst for large samples and averaging statistics, it ignores the nuance and neglects the subtleties of the individual subjective impression. It is here where artists and the practice of art can be so valuable in bringing alive what crass people, in everyday life, may always have scorned and suppressed.

Recovery axiomatically is a longitudinal concept so what is helpful tends to vary over time as one develops and changes. In my situation I only was ready to return to work after two years and full-time work was only possible after about five years. I was only ready to apply depth psychological approaches to myself after about five years and, as I said above, in the immediate aftermath of the crisis a very practical here-and-now approach was best so as gradually to enculture me back into society. One has to re-learn how to see people and the world – in an everyday sense – as everybody else does, rather than perceiving everything through the lens of a spectacular delusion – and most delusions do tend to be spectacular, as if the person is trying to extract from life more than life really has to give.

It is in some respects a shock, even a disappointment, to rejoin the mundane, everyday world but that is where one has to re-learn how to find one's meaning and purpose. This is not something one can do very quickly, patience and the willingness to take things gradually and not to be too upset by setbacks, are all vital.

It is important that professionals do not see patients and clients only through the lenses of their own pet theories and approaches as the diversity of people at the individual level is the very essence of the human world. Working with statistical averages all the time can blind professionals to this. Therapy sessions may need to be inordinately long or indeed short and the use of extraordinarily intense eye contact ('the therapeutic stare') is not to be recommended with recovering psychotic clients – nor is directly facing seats. One has to be sensitive to the existing schemata and mental models people already have there in their heads to which to attach new information and strategies. It is no use if both client and professional are talking their own private language, 'joint reference' is absolutely essential, otherwise the whole experience of dealing with the professional induces a strange feeling of utter alienation ('I'm in my world, he's in his world, between us is Nothingness'). Jean-Paul Sartre would give a wry smile.

Professionals also need to be exceedingly wary of showing the same cognitive biases as the patients, such as confirmation bias and jumping to conclusions. Overenthusiastic use of diagnostic categories and psychological clichés often prompts such processes in professionals, it is lamentable when one sees this happen.

One has to recognise that since recovery to a meaningful and fulfilling life is itself a life process, there is bound to be a 'horses for courses' element to all this and sufferers will need to do some 'conceptual shopping,' as I call it, to see which avenues are, at any one time, likely to be the most fruitful and stimulating for them. In my case the concepts of Gestalt therapy and Person-Centred therapy were always extremely helpful and thought provoking – despite the fact that neither of these approaches has any great track record in the treatment of psychosis. Not everybody, of course, temperamentally is suited to cognitive procedures (where the stronger evidence base lies) but many cognitive professionals do incorporate ideas and techniques from Gestalt and Person-Centred therapies into their skills repertoire (see Freeman, Bentall and Garety, 2008).

Recovery is a creative, individual and developmental process. It is not something to be engineered in a machine-like way, as the vicissitudes of life only permit thinking like that to be effective to a local, limited degree. Really, in essence, it is an adventure and a challenge in which the future is revealed and constructed as we probe. But certainly the more interpretive resources, life and social skills, insights and perceptions one can amass, the better one will be prepared for the fluctuations of fortune that are all inevitable aspects of the journey in time we all have before us on this earth.

From calumny to stillness

As one might expect, my own decadent journey – at least when I was much younger - prompted ridicule, contempt, gossip and rumour-spreading, insults, sneers, occasional violent assaults and eventually insanity and suicide attempts. Now the war in my life and in my head is over and in my seventh decade I have the peacefulness of a rather 'teddy bear' personality. It's not really masculine *or* feminine but both and neither. This integration is how it should be. Alas, some doctors, however, don't expect me to live even another two years. It has all taken its toll on my physical health, particularly my heart, even if within, mentally, my mind is, at least now, placid and free from strife. Still: one should aim to look back on one's life as having been a worthwhile progression. The psychoanalyst Erik Erikson knew this. This I do. Currently I have also to look forward, however, to the afterlife. This is the next challenge. And..... you know what? I think it will be *very* interesting to have a talk with my father.

References

Bebbington, P. and McGuffin, P. (Eds) (1988) *Schizophrenia: The Major Issues.* London: Heinemann.

Chadwick, P.K. (1979) Understanding Transvestism. *The World of Transvestism,* 1(8): 33-5.

Chadwick, P. K. (1992) *Borderline: A psychological study of paranoia and delusional thinking,* London: Routledge.

Chadwick, P. K. (1993) The stepladder to the impossible: A first hand phenomenological account of a schizoaffective psychotic crisis. *Journal of Mental Health,* 2: 239-50.

Chadwick, P. K. (1995a) The artist as psychologist. *The Psychologist* (Letters), 8(9): 391.

Chadwick, P. K. (1995b) In search of deep music: Artistic approaches to the study of mind. *Clinical Psychology Forum,* 89 (March): 8-11.

Chadwick, P. K. (1997a) Transvestism: A psychologist's view, *The World of Transvestism,* 18(11): 14-22.

Chadwick, P. K. (1997b) Recovery from psychosis – Learning more from patients. *Journal of Mental Health,* 6, 6, 577-88.

Chadwick, P. K. (2001a) Psychotic consciousness. *International Journal of Social Psychiatry,* 47(1): 52-62.

Chadwick, P. K. (2001b) Sanity to supersanity to insanity: A personal journey, in I. Clarke (ed) *Psychosis and Spirituality: Exploring the New Frontier.* London: Whurr.

Chadwick, P. K. (2001c) *Personality as Art: Artistic approaches in psychology.* Ross-on-Wye: PCCS Books.

Chadwick, P. K. (2003) The stream of psychotic consciousness, *Open Mind,* 124: 22-3.

Chadwick, P. K. (2006a) Oscar Wilde: The playwright as psychologist. *The Wildean,* 28: 17-23.

Chadwick, P. K. (2006b) On the masculinity and heterosexuality thought police (MASHTOP). *The Journal of Critical Psychology Counselling and Psychotherapy,* 6 (4): 200-209.

Chadwick, P. K. (2007a) Freud meets Wilde: A playlet. *The Wildean,* 31: 2-22.

Chadwick, P. K. (2007b) On the dominance of male metaphors for thought in psychology. *The Journal of Critical Psychology, Counselling and Psychotherapy,* 7(3): 146-9.

Chadwick, P. K. (2008) *Schizophrenia – The Positive Perspective: Explorations at the Outer Reaches of Human Experience.* London: Routledge.

Freeman, D., Bentall, R. and Garety, P. (2008) *Persecutory Delusions: Assessment, Theory and*

Treatment. Oxford: Oxford University Press.

Garety, P. and Freeman, D. (1999) Cognitive approaches to delusions: A critical review of theories and evidence. *British Journal of Clinical Psychology,* 38 (2): 113-54.

Gergen, K.J. (1990) Therapeutic professions and the diffusion of deficit. *Journal of Mind and Behaviour,* 11, 353-67.

Laing, R.D. (1960) *The Divided Self.* London: Tavistock.

Rogers, C.R. (1961) *On Becoming a Person.* Boston: Houghton Mifflin.

Rogers, C. R. (1980) *A Way of Being,* Boston: Houghton Mifflin.

Wason, P.C. (1960) On the failure to eliminate hypotheses in a conceptual task. *Quarterly Journal of Experimental Psychology,* 12:129-140.

9

Does a psychotic episode ever do anybody any good?

Peter K. Chadwick

In his second chapter, Peter starts by looking at the economic costs of schizophrenia. This is not to mention the huge psychological costs both for the sufferers and their families. Peter asks the question, 'What if anything is to be gained by the experience of having a psychotic episode?' He argues that there is a need for more positive narratives, 'We do after all need discourses that are helpful to people, not discourses that demoralise them.' Peter gives one example of an artist called Aidan Shingler. While Aidan reports having had 13 psychotic episodes and three hospital admissions, he claims that his psychotic experiences were growth periods and evidence of increased psychic sensitivity. He claims to have been able to turn his psychotic experiences into art works. Peter also gives the example of Mad Pride, which tries to put a positive framework on psychotic experiences. Yet, Peter challenges what he feels is a lack of personal responsibility in some of its advocates and as he mentions in the previous chapter, almost a disregard for the effects of madness on those closest to the sufferer. Peter is in no doubt that his own psychotic experience was a positive for him, and that he went onto achieve a great deal following his own psychotic crisis. Medication had, and continues to play, a significant part in his own recovery.

Schizophrenia: The dark side

Schizophrenia affects at least 24 million people worldwide and the WHO lists it as the second largest contributor to the overall burden of disease, after cardiovascular disease. Treatment of schizophrenia alone costs 34 billion dollars in the USA in 2001, almost a third of all mental healthcare spending. Average life expectancy of sufferers is reduced by 10 years, 30-60% attempt suicide at least once in a lifetime and about 10%-12% die from suicide.

The illness is associated with immense emotional and physical costs to sufferers and their families, there is impaired social functioning and about half have a co-morbid substance use disorder, while 80% of older patients have a co-morbid physical disorder. Schizophrenia sufferers also are more likely to be arrested and charged with a crime and the illness causes high rates of unemployment not only in sufferers but in many carers as well. All of these difficulties cause increased burden and lost productivity (Samnaliev and Clark, 2011). Costs of schizophrenia treatment in the UK were estimated at £2.6 billion by Knapp (1997 – see also Essock, Frisman and Covell, 2003) but there are now sharply escalating costs of the more expensive atypical or second generation antipsychotic medications which may absorb as much as 90% of actual medication costs. Between 1996 and 2001 the price increase in the USA was 77%. In 2004 antipsychotic drug expenditure there reached 20 billion dollars.

The indirect costs of family caregiving are much more difficult to quantify. Parents not only shoulder immense emotional burden but also give financial assistance to schizophrenia sufferers, as much as twice as much as to other children. Family members therefore may actually decrease costs of formal mental healthcare.

In a scenario as grim as this, I think it is important to consider the other side of the coin and ask what sufferers actually get out of a psychotic episode, if anything, to nourish them on the rest of their journey through life. One recent study, for example, (Cordle, Fradgley, Carson, Holloway and Richards, 2011) suggests, surprisingly, that the picture might not be all so negative.

Patients' reflections

Narratives in Cordle *et al.* do show that for some sufferers, the crisis and their recovery efforts have given them more understanding of themselves and indeed have helped them find out who they really are. One sees this in the accounts of Michelle McNary (p.82 in Cordle *et al.*); Stuart Baker-Brown (p.192); Peter Bullimore (p.162); Gordon McManus (p.132) and Helen George (p.122). On more specific issues, psychosis can be seen as a profound creative and spiritual experience (Emma Harding, pp.142-3) and/or as a means of enhancing creativity (Stuart Baker-Brown, p.192) or as giving the person new ways of thinking about their art (Ben Haydon, pp.91-2).

In other respects James Bellamy feels that the whole psychotic experience has made him less selfish and more willing to help and assist others (p.112) while others have found that the crisis has helped clarify or strengthen their spirituality (Esther Maxwell-Orumbie, p.172; Carl Lee, pp.150-1; Helen George, p.122). Sufferers may speak of money being now less important in their lives (Peter Bullimore, p.162; Bose Dania, p.102) and of feeling more positive towards themselves, secure and grounded (Carl Lee, pp.150-1; Peter Bullimore, p.162; Helen George, p.122).

These strengthening and positive discourses are, of course, not unique to one text. See also Clarke (2010) and Basset and Stickley (2010). Author and playwright Des Marshall (see Marshall, 2002; Chadwick, 2008) who was tottering on the very edge of psychosis in 1992 has recovered particularly by utilising the healing powers of creativity (in his case, writing) and spirituality (see Lukoff, 2010, also on the latter). Des prefers not to define spirituality but simply leaves it as that which helps him to be loving, compassionate, forgiving, more open to the world and better able to relate to people. Since 1992 he has come to feel more equal to people, less of an Outsider and less prone to tantrums.

From these accounts, and others (see, for example, Chadwick, 1992, and the strengths-based approach to case management in Rapp and Goscha, 2011) one can see that focussing on positive qualities in psychosis sufferers is empowering and hope-giving. We do, after all, need discourses that are helpful to people, not discourses that demoralise them. Some sufferers, of course, angry and demeaned by the deficit, dysfunction and diagnosis-driven nature of much psychosis research, have attempted to reclaim the schizophrenic experience for themselves rather than have it seen as an illness and hence as a category apart. One recent attempt to explore the spiritual and creative potential of schizophrenia is that of Shingler (2008).

Schizophrenia as art and spirituality

Shingler's text 'One in a hundred' was reviewed as 'inexplicably beautiful' by *The Guardian* and 'A shaft of light into the darkness' by *Arts Journal*. In it he tries to see schizophrenia as an 'evolutionary metamorphosis' leading to a state of enlightenment. To him, schizophrenia is more a spiritual conflict than an illness (p.14) and he argues that it has the potential – as we have seen here previously – to enhance creativity and develop the personality positively (p.12). He claims (p.77) to have integrated and understood his experiences and resolved them and that his episodes have helped him to comprehend himself 'in relation to this Earthly and Universal Adventure' (p.78).

Although he adopts the less controversial position (p.12) of saying that schizophrenia can broaden perspectives and perceptions he also claims that schizophrenia sufferers are receptive to the paranormal. I have to say that in my experience, with reference to relating the metaphysical and the paranormal to psychosis, the only people that this means a lot to tends to be the patients themselves who have, like myself, actually 'been there'. The amplification of the uncanny and the increase in frequency of the synchronistic mean something to the patients but are meaningless to the professionals – who dismiss such talk without seriously listening as 'illness talk' or as 'hippy 1960s talk'. There is, of course, some experimental evidence confirmatory of enhancement of paranormal sensitivities in psychosis (Lee, 1991, 1994) but stressing this does seem to actually destabilise people. In one study (see Greyson, 1977) some participants actually found the *negative* outcome, of a test of paranormal capacities in psychosis, therapeutic. So this, clearly, is a double-edged sword and the proposition has to be handled carefully.

There seems, however, little doubt that Shingler's *perception* of schizophrenia has helped him. He presents his 13 psychotic episodes as growth experiences towards enlightenment and rejects psychiatry's construction of schizophrenia as damaging of the journey to enlightenment.

His is an altered state of consciousness which he seems to have maintained not as a state at all but as a disposition. It is rare that people can do this for such a length of time, in Shingler's case decades. His actual psychotic episodes he talks of as 'psychic openings' not psychotic episodes at all.

An atmosphere of a certain degree of euphoria pervades the text. It is an uplifting frame of mind which he has put to artistic use, turning what a professional in the human sciences would see as symptoms into artistic images and installations. His disposition, if not psychotic, is what most professionals would see as borderline. He is extra-sensitive to coincidences and, for example, sees cosmic meanings in Milky Way chocolate bars and a Wisdom toothbrush. But, again, Shingler doesn't leave it at that but turns these perceptions into art.

Most professionals wouldn't see 13 psychotic episodes and three hospitalisations as signalling increasing resolution of his experiences as he claims on p.77. Still, to him they are growth experiences, evidence of psychic sensitivity, not madness at all. He has, however, certainly made art out of what most people would interpret as psychosis and has presented it not as an inferior form of art. This of course is parallel and supplementary to previous work which sees art by psychosis sufferers as having its own validity and dignity and being worthy of the title of art in its own right (e.g. MacGregor, 1989; Prinzhorn, 1995).

The scientific community in psychiatry and abnormal psychology adopts for the most part a realist position in ideological terms which enables it to claim 'truth' via the evidence of the senses. In an increasingly post-modern world, such a position is seen as itself only one (power-seeking) construction that can be put on human life and on how to study it. In a social constructionist scenario (Gergen, 1985; 1990) many other perspectives are possible (including Shingler's) deriving from different assumptions about reality and our place as perceivers and interpreters of 'The World'. In mental health such perspectives are producing texts which seriously challenge realist discourses on the academic stage (e.g. Stone, 2006; Sparkes and Douglas, 2007; Carless and Douglas, 2010). Emboldened by arguments that see reality as socially constructed rather than as externally 'there' to be perceived by a disinterested, dispassionate observer taking 'objective' measurements, many investigators and interest groups are now exploring other possible ways of seeking knowledge and influencing policy and practice. Given the disastrous ways that the realist researchers have behaved in their studies of women, black people and gays, such people – indeed like Shingler – have reclaimed themselves away from the identity of 'objects for objective study' (usually by white, male, middle class scientists) to reclaim their experiences, as he has done, as intrinsically valid in their own terms. In the context of mental health in the UK, the actual organisation that has blossomed along these lines is, of course, *Mad Pride* (Curtis, Dellar, Leslie and Watson, 2000).

Psychosis as positive-in-itself: *Mad Pride*

Mad Pride see the positivity of psychosis as imbricated there *in* the psychosis itself, not a feature of its aftermath or of the recovery process. For example on p.207 of Curtis *et al.* we find: 'There really is so much that's positive and exciting about 'illnesses' like 'schizophrenia'. All of us who've experienced 'deep sea fishing' will know the sensation of heightened awareness, of consciousness enhanced far better than LSD ever could do it, of feelings of wonder and terror that can't be verbalised... and then have these visions which effortlessly outstrip the alienation of daily life dismissed as 'delusion' by some fucking shrink. Nearly everything that's 'bad' about madness is caused by the reactions of the restrained, shrivelled and grey majority to someone near them being beautifully crazy and alive!' (Simon Morris, 2000, p.207).

In the book the various authors write from the perspective of just being *with* their insanity and seek the liberation and intrinsic validity of mad people free of coercion and abusive therapeutic techniques. In firecracker prose that is alternately rational, poetic and, at times, just mind-scrambling, there is much accusation directed at bourgeois capitalism and the alienated individualism of the success-striving, 9-5 existence as insanity inducing and a colourful thrust for freedom from the chains, demands and restrictions imposed by social agents. But there is little on the day-to-day responsibilities of psychosis experiencers (e.g. Chadwick, 2010) and little about consideration for other people whose lives are made chaotic, even wrecked, by mad behaviour. A murder by a psychotic (p.125) is passed over with little comment as if it's 'all in the game'. The term 'social conscience' appears just once in the book, on p.114. The claim is that madness has to be reclaimed from scientists and is the new rock n'roll – which is a variant of the general modernist ideology whose basic bottom line is '...... so let's have fun'. And if we end up killing ourselves, even by disembowelment (p.213) then so be it. Too bad. Our job, like rock stars, is to change the world so it's easier, in which, for people like us to live.

Acknowledging the rather adolescent tone of all this, for me there is no doubt, however, that madness has liberating aspects. In my own case my mind became less dry and tight and so more supple after the episode and I discovered the value and power of fiction making in the short stories I wrote (see Chapter 8) whereas previously I had been chained only to fact and a very arid style of objective reason. I also accessed and intensified my underdeveloped spiritual side (Chapter 8) with experiences that I have learned from and never forgotten. And I am someone whose episode turned out to be horrific, not beautiful and is something of which I am definitely not proud nor something in which I in any way rejoice.

So the deep core of the *Mad Pride* message seems to me to have some validity, or at least *can* be valid. What this civil liberties movement needs is the balance provided by recognition of the responsibilities that increased freedom always bring and recognition of the rights, importance and dignity of carers and befrienders who seemingly are mere ghosts of the solipsistic in *Mad Pride* consciousness.

Up then down, down then up

It often, if not always, is the case that the euphoria associated particularly with mania, hypomania and some schizoaffective episodes can firstly make psychosis temporarily rewarding but the clash with the societal requirement to have consideration for other people then crumbles the positivity to rubble. One patient with unipolar mania painted the toilet area in his hostel in bright colours when he was 'high', certainly improving its appearance, but also punched one of the female social workers in the stomach in the same state – shouting 'Have some respect for your elders!' This was a serious downside, particularly considering that the social worker was pregnant.

Similarly one hypomanic patient noticed, at three o'clock in the morning, that the floorboards in his flat were not aligned quite right – so he decided to lever them up and nail them back so that they fitted together more accurately. Perhaps his flooring was improved while everybody in the house was kept awake all night. He was sectioned.

Many people do find the psychotic state exciting and uplifting such that when self-inflatory spectacular delusions collapse, they are precipitated into a post-psychotic depression sometimes made worse by the zombie state induced by the medication. One man said that when he was ill he had the power to look at a sick person and when he looked away their illness was 'taken away' from them. Another likened being ill to visiting Mars while the return to the sane state was like 'going to work in a fish and chip shop' by comparison. Another admitted that deep down she knew that she was 'kidding herself' when deluded, but kept the game up for the excitement.

One has to admit, even as a former sufferer myself, that the euphoria of insanity, if it obtains, is a Janus-faced entity. Its high intensity can easily transmute, as the cues change, into feelings of damnation, threat, antagonism and/or self-hatred all at continued and maintained intensity. All altered states of consciousness seem to have this duplex quality. It is the price to be paid for departing from the realm of everyday sobriety. Travellers into altered states seek a holiday for the mind but go with no guarantees or insurance.

I wonder though to what extent psychosis is an *adventure?* Does one seek, as with illicit drugs, one altered state too many? Does one look for an antidote to boredom only to end up confronting one's deepest fears and inadequacies? Can psychosis be a necessary confrontation as so many report it has been? A date with one's deepest Self? This puts quite a different complexion on it to just seeing it as meaningless derangement and dysfunction.

Some people do feel that madness 'boiled something out of their system' such as a wildly overoptimistic ambition (realised only in insanity and then dispensed with) or a terrible dread they've always feared (at last confronted in insanity). Recovery seems to have been rather better in people who talk like that about their episode. It seems to have genuinely made them able to move on, even if sadder but wiser.

It is evident that 'down then up' themes are not totally missing from the biographies of psychosis sufferers. The discovery of poetry and art-making after psychosis is, of course, quite a common theme in the mental health culture. It turns the material released to consciousness into something shareable and is a way therefore of actually communicating it.

Most people find communication of the psychotic state itself incredibly difficult – as dream recall and communication often is. Art and poetry therefore act here as conduits from the personal to the public and hence partake of the healing power of communication and meaning-making. This may also be related to the possibility of psychosis making neural networks more associatively 'supple' without automatically or necessarily making them forever 'loose'.

The 'down then up' scenario is, of course, reminiscent also of R.D. Laing's claim (Laing 1960, 1967) that the 'schizophrenic voyage', if left to run to completion, can leave you better than you were before. This is a view, however, not unique to Laing. Silverman (1967, 1970) argues that the Laingian scenario can be lived out and *is* lived out to completion particularly in some cultures of a very different spiritual climate to that of the West – at least when the crisis has strong spiritual accompaniments. Then the sufferer is not seen as 'an acute schizophrenic' by the community but comes to be seen, on resolution of the crisis, as a healer and shaman and their status is elevated not diminished. That psychosis can be a transition to a spiritually more developed state was also a view pioneered by Boisen (1947, 1952) while the positive relationships between the mystical and the psychotic have been pointed out by Lenz (1979) and Heriot-Maitland (2008). Both Silverman (1967) and Heriot-Maitland (2008) explicitly see mystical and psychotic states as involving similar psychological processes. To Silverman the essential difference between the two lies in the degree of cultural acceptance and support of the individual's psychological resolution of a life crisis (p.23). He writes that 'such supports are all too often completely unavailable to the schizophrenic in our culture' (p.29).

Silverman (1970, p.63) quotes Karl Menninger who said in 1959, 'Some patients have a mental illness and then get well and then they get weller! I mean they get better than they ever were.... This is an extraordinary and little realised truth'. Whether in our culture such 'positive disintegration' can lead to impressive reorganisation and personal growth is as controversial today (for example in the work of Rufus May 2000; 2006) as it was in the 1960s and 1970s. Silverman was optimistic in 1970 but time has generally favoured, at least in the West, a more 'interfering' approach to the development of psychotic states. Certainly my own crisis was resolved with the *aid*, not the hindrance, of medication yet I am certainly better than I ever was. So the two approaches may not be as disjunctive as Laing and Silverman made them out to be. Of the people I have known who are better now than they ever were, about half have benefitted from small doses of medication (Chadwick, 2002, p.12).

Conclusions

The discourses that people are encapsulated within on admission to mental health services can make their situation worse, not better. It does seem, however, that psychosis can enable people to make gains, not losses, in their journey through life. It is important that the person finds or creates a discourse that fits their situation and needs and it is likely that this will involve some 'conceptual shopping' particularly in their early months and years of recovery. Perhaps the key word here is 'flexibility' on the part of service user and professional. Sufferers do however seem to find positive discourses particularly helpful (Martyn, 2002) rather than being forced to see themselves as a mass of deficits and dysfunctions. At the present stage of our knowledge it does seem as if a post-modern approach utilising many different perspectives from which to choose, is the best way ahead. This should not however aggressively pre-empt, for some people, more conventional or indeed more outré, approaches

References

Basset, T. & Stickley, T. (2010) (eds), *Voices of Experience: Narratives of Mental Health Survivors*. Chichester: Wiley.

Boisen, A.T. (1947) Onset in acute psychosis. *Psychiatry*, 10, 159-67.

Boisen, A.T. (1952) Mystical identification in mental disorder. *Psychiatry*, 15, 287-97.

Carless, D. & Douglas, K. (2010) *Sport and Physical Activity for Mental Health*. Chichester: Wiley-Blackwell.

Chadwick, P.K. (1992) *Borderline: A psychological study of paranoia and delusional thinking*. London: Routledge.

Chadwick, P.K. (2002) How to become better after psychosis than you were before. *Open Mind*, 115 (May/June), 12-13.

Chadwick, P.K. (2008) *Schizophrenia, the Positive Perspective (Second edition): Explorations at the Outer Reaches of Human Experience.* London: Routledge.

Chadwick, P.K. (2010) Taking responsibility for one's mental illness: Advantages and difficulties. *British Journal of Wellbeing*, 1(9)(December), 10-12.

Clarke, I., (2010) ed., *Psychosis and Spirituality (Second edition): Consolidating the New Paradigm.* Chichester: Wiley.

Cordle, H., Fradgley, J., Carson, J., Holloway, F. & Richards, P. (2011) *Psychosis: Stories of Recovery and Hope.* London: Quay Books.

Curtis, T., Dellar, R., Leslie, E. & Watson, B. (2000) *Mad Pride: A Celebration of Mad Culture.* London: Spare Change Books.

Essock, S.M., Frisman, L.K. & Covell, N.H. (2003) Economics of the treatment of schizophrenia. In S.R. Hirsch and D.R. Weinberger, *Schizophrenia* (Second Edition). Oxford, Massachusetts: Blackwell Science.

Gergen, K.J. (1985) The social constructionist movement in modern psychology. *American Psychologist*, 40, 266-75.

Gergen, K.J. (1990) Therapeutic professions and the diffusion of deficit. *Journal of Mind and Behaviour*, 11, 353-67.

Greyson, B. (1977) Telepathy in mental illness: deluge or delusion? *Journal of Nervous and Mental Disease*, 165, 184-200.

Heriot-Maitland, C.P. (2008) Mysticism and madness: different aspects of the same human experience? *Mental Health, Religion and Culture*, 11, 301-25.

Knapp, M. (1997) Costs of schizophrenia. *British Journal of Psychiatry*, 171, 509-18.

Laing, R.D. (1960) *The Divided Self.* London: Penguin.

Laing, R.D. (1967) *The Politics of Experience and The Bird of Paradise.* London: Penguin.

Lee, A.G. (1991) About the investigation technique of some unusual mental phenomena. *Parapsychology in the USSR*, 2, 34-8.

Lee, A.G. (1994) Extrasensory phenomena in the psychiatric clinic. *Parapsychology and Psychophysics*, 1, 53-6.

Lenz, H. (1979) The element of the irrational at the beginning and during the course of delusion. *Confinia Psychiatrica*, 22, 183-90.

Lukoff, D. (2010) Visionary spiritual experiences. In I. Clarke (ed), *Psychosis and Spirituality: Consolidating the New Paradigm.* Chichester: Wiley.

MacGregor, J.M. (1989) *The Discovery of the Art of the Insane.* Princeton, N.J.: Princeton University Press.

Marshall, D. (2002) *Journal of an Urban Robinson Crusoe: London and Brighton.* Burgess Hill, West Sussex: Saxon Books.

Martyn, D. (2002) *The Experiences and Views of Self-Management of People with a Schizophrenia Diagnosis.* London: NSF Self Management Project.

May, R. (2000) Routes to recovery from psychosis: the roots of a clinical psychologist. *Clinical Psychology Forum*, 146, 6-10.

May, R. (2006) Resisting the diagnostic gaze. *Journal of Critical Psychology, Counselling and Psychotherapy*, 6(3), 155-8.

Morris, S. (2000) Heaven is a mad place on earth. In T. Curtis, R. Dellar, E. Leslie and B. Watson (eds) *Mad Pride: A Celebration of Mad Culture*. London: Spare Change Books.

Prinzhorn, H. (1995) *Artistry of the Mentally Ill* (translated by Eric Von Brockdorff,). New York: Springer Verlag.

Rapp, C.A. & Gosha, R.J. (2011) Strengths-based case management. In K.T. Mueser and D.V. Jeste (eds) *Clinical Handbook of Schizophrenia*. New York: The Guilford Press.

Samnaliev, M. & Clarke, R.E. (2011) The economics of schizophrenia. In K.T. Mueser and D.V. Jeste (eds) *Clinical Handbook of Schizophrenia*. New York: The Guilford Press.

Shingler, A. (2008) *One in a Hundred*. Wirksworth, Derbyshire: Thorntree Press.

Silverman, J. (1967) Shamans and acute schizophrenia. *American Anthropologist*, 69, 21-31.

Silverman, J. (1970) When schizophrenia helps. *Psychology Today*, 4 (September), 63-70.

Sparkes, A.C. & Douglas, K. (2007) Making the case for poetic representations: An example in action. *Sport Psychologist*, 21(2), 170-189.

Stone, B. (2006) Diaries, self talk and psychosis: Writing as a place to live. *Auto/ Biography*, 14, 41-58.

10

Recovery: What I have learned from my own journey of Recovery

Dolly Sen

Dolly Sen has been a pioneer in the service user recovery movement in South London. Her chapter starts with the distressing image of her poised, ready to strike, with a knife above the sleeping form of her father. Seeing a photograph of herself as a young child on the wall miraculously stops her from committing patricide. She tells us how she got to this position from a childhood of abuse. Her psychosis started with persecutory voices from the age of 14. Then one day she made the momentous decision to transform her life. She had to stop relying on psychiatry to find the cure. She realised she had to do it for herself. 'Recovery for me was and is creating...Moving from insanity to being sane is moving from one world to another and is pretty scary.' Dolly then gives us her tips and tools that she used on her own recovery journey, such as positivity and having goals. She lists what she feels were the significant points that helped propel her life forward. She states, 'I want to leave a legacy to say: Dolly Sen was here.' She concludes her account with the inspirational statement, 'What I know about recovery is that the more you believe it is possible, the more you will recover.'

A note to mental health professionals

Recovery is not a prescription given to a patient by a doctor. Recovery is a letter of hopes, dreams, songs, peace, hurt, chaos, transcendence, night and light given to the mental health professional by the patient. Read it and believe in it. Let it be a map. Maybe you will be only the painter of signposts, but to help somebody on the way back to their heart, is the way to go to yours.

This is my map, this is the way back to my own heart.

Life before recovery

'I'm self-hate surrounded by mirrors. Not the many glass ones I have shattered, ensuring I have no good luck for the next thousand lifetimes. No, the mirror of the eyes that constantly watch me. Mirrors with names, smiles, souls and lies.

'You've got your Daddy's eyes and your Daddy's lies. Cut them out!' The voices tell me over and over again.

Can memories turn into psychosis? These are memories that touch me with the insistence of a branding iron. Writing this memoir, I have to make sure that it doesn't turn into a suicide note.

My father was an actor and musician, so I grew up in the entertainment industry. My father also thought of himself as a comedian, but you didn't hear much laughter in our home.

The first film I remember working in as an extra was 'The Empire Strikes Back'. The film set was the interior of a space station and there were all kinds of monsters walking about. I didn't know it was make-believe – I thought it was a documentary. 20 years later my mind had left planet Earth too.

'You've got your Daddy's eyes and your Daddy's lies. Cut them out!'

I'm standing over my sleeping father with a knife in my hand. Because he is a demonic alien plotting my destruction, he has to die; I am going to bring down the knife down on his face. 'Look who's laughing now,' I say. It doesn't matter to me that I am heading for a special hospital or eventual suicide. As a mental health professional said to me: 'Dolly, your next stop is Broadmoor.' It didn't matter because I did what I had to do to survive. Can't people understand that?

As he sleeps, I watch him, waiting for the right moment to kill. Waiting. Waiting. His awful body odour, the old food in his beard, the spit marks on the floor, just makes me angrier and angrier. I raise the knife, ready to plunge it into this waste of a human being. Another set of eyes is staring at me - from the wall. It is a picture of me as a child, smiling for the camera. I try three times to stab my father's skull, but a child is watching, and I can't do it. 'I'm sorry for turning you into a murderer,' I say to the photo. 'I used to be a child once, I used to be a little girl...'

This is how I start my mental health memoir 'The World is Full of Laughter.' That moment described was the culmination of decades of abuse at the hands of my father and his friends, and several years of psychosis and depression. It was the worst point in my life. It had to be if I wanted to kill my father to ease my pain. But strangely enough it was also the beginning of my recovery, because something did click. As I looked at the photo of me as a child, I realised I couldn't let that child live this kind of life. Something had to change. But what of that child?

Life before psychosis

At aged 14 I had already gone through what most people don't suffer in a lifetime. Physical, emotional, mental, sexual abuse, racism, poverty, neglect, bullying, and more. Most importantly there wasn't any hope. I learnt very early to become hopeless in order to protect myself. I remember only having 3 hopes as a child: one, to be loved; two, not to be abused; and thirdly, to have a bicycle. 'You'll get one when you're good,' Dad promised. Birthdays and Christmases came and went – no bike year upon year upon year. All I wanted was a bike. Seeing other kids riding their own bikes made me so jealous. Just imagine being promised something you really want 1001 times, and not getting it 1001 times. Soon I stopped wanting ... anything.

No hope. No hope. Was it any wonder I cracked under the strain? In my book *The World is Full of Laughter* I say of my time directly before my breakdown, I had:

> A brace in a mouth that didn't know how to or want to talk.
> Shoes from Tesco.
> A bra that didn't fit.
> Knickers that had holes in them.
> A body bruised.
> A body touched by dirty old men
> And ignored by the rest of the world.
> I was beginning to lose my mind...

My experience of psychosis

The first auditory hallucination I recall happened around about this time; I was 14. Every Sunday the radio would play the UK top 40. I listened to it and taped the songs I liked. All of a sudden the music went quiet and a troll-like voice issued from the radio: 'What do you want, Dolly? How much do you want?' My skin prickled. I shut off the radio in fear. Deep demonic laughter followed. 'Can't get rid of me. I'm yours for life now.' 'Who are you?' 'I am the universe. I choose whether you live or breathe.' I got up and ran out of the room. I stopped listening to the radio from then on. As the days passed, I thought maybe I just dreamed it all. The voices then chose the TV as their medium. I was drowning in a sea of bad ads that I had to read into for cosmic significance. Soon I stopped watching TV. I became obsessed with the battle between good and evil played out in 'The Empire Strikes Back.' I was thinking: Everybody thinks it is just a film, entertaining make-believe, but that was what *they* wanted you to think. But *that* was the reality, and the audience watching and their little lives was the fantasy.

Stress increased the hallucinations and delusions. One time Dad pressed my hand down on the oven hob; the skin of my hand sizzled and throbbed. Holding my burning hand, I ran into my bedroom. I had a picture of Jesus on the wall. I looked up at it and begged him to help me. He just stared blankly down at me, his bleeding palms facing me. Our hands looked similar. I understood then I was being persecuted for being Jesus by the demon that was my father. He wanted me to die. He was behind the voices that told me to jump down a stairwell. When I was on the street, they told me to step into oncoming traffic.

There was also depression and its associated negative thinking: 'I can't do anything right. Why do people move away from me on the bus? I must smell or be so horrifically ugly people can't take being on the same planet as me. Stop laughing at me, Satan! Stop laughing at me, God! It says a lot about life that the Devil and God laugh at the same thing. Nobody loves me, not even my family. They wish I were dead and out of their lives. I am evil and contaminate anything that looks at me. I can't do anything right. Why am I letting myself live? The pain in my body is too big for my skin, maybe I should cut it open and let it all seep out. I want to cut the eyes out of my head so the world won't hurt as much. Nobody loves me. Would death even want me or would it spit me out like a bad seed? I should kill myself, what's the point in living like this? I want to die but I'm too scared to. See, I can't do anything right. I am evil, evil, evil, evil, evil, evil. Please, God, Don't let me wake up to another horrible day. I can't do anything right. Every second of my life I regret. The future will only promise more regrets and more instances to exercise cowardice. Mum should have had an abortion...' This caustic commentary I listened to every night for hours on end until I was exhausted enough to sleep. They were there when I woke up, paralysing me so much I was incapable of lifting my head off the pillow.

All this accumulated into the moment where I stood over my father with a knife. It was a moment full of horror but there was a flash of overwhelming grace: I knew I had to change. There and then I made the decision to work on my recovery. I dropped the knife and never picked it up again.

The first steps towards recovery

But I didn't know how to change, so I looked – not to psychiatry – but to my interest in Buddhism to show me ways to change. I threw myself into Buddhist practice. Meditation de-stressed me, made me a calmer person. It also helped me challenge low self-esteem's mantra of: 'I cannot do this' or 'I'm not worth it'. I was no longer going to let a sentence that doesn't even last 3 seconds dictate the whole of my life. I utilised the trick of looking upon each day as my last day of life, and filled it with good things.

So one of the things I did was to go the Grand Canyon for a holiday. I wasn't disappointed. The magnitude of its beauty brought tears to my eyes. There was no doubt it was bigger than any human being, greater than any God. The changing sun transformed the colours of the rock and brought them alive. It may be just a tourist attraction for some, but for me it was a changing point in my life: I could no longer completely believe in suicide any more, not when life could give me this. I was one step from the edge of the cliff, and the stunning view stopped me in my tracks; I was unable to take another step.

I had the inspiration to change, but of course things were not plain-sailing. You have to account for the loss of identity with regards to psychosis. Psychosis touches your heart, mind, and soul, and turns it all in on itself, like a knot that has no beginning or end. It turns your life into a ghost train ride without end, haunted by spectres and on the edge of your seat with fear for what seems like forever. Imagine a nightmare so horrible you have to open your eyes. But guess what? What you open your eyes to is even worse, more monsters, more fear. Close your eyes, open them, close your eyes, open them. No respite. Identity is lost in that blink of an eye.

So you go to the psychiatrist and they give you a label. Schizophrenia? Manic Depression? You become a set of symptoms. You become the illness. Everything else does not exist. Your childhood, your aspirations, your dreams, your likes and dislikes, your quirks and sense of humour become meaningless. Every time you see a mental health professional, they say 'What's wrong with *you*?' Anything else about your life is of no interest to them. So is it any wonder that an already fragile identity is lost? If you are your illness, what is the point of hope?

I have taken my pill, so now what? My heart is still breaking, my childhood still broken. My dreams are still in my head. THEY say I am not allowed to dream them. That I have no right, it will make me too big for my boots. Don't get above your station. THEY say I am not capable of dreaming or making those dreams come true. My prognosis clearly states: 'No dreams, no dreams allowed'. To find dreams in the midst of the nightmare that is paranoia, depression, delusions of evil, and horrible, tormenting voices is hard. That is a journey in itself, and I think I spent a decade of my life (my 20s) doing just that. But no matter: I say screw you. I WILL dream. Your pills won't stop me dreaming. I will leave you behind. My heart WILL heal. With or without you.

That was another thing that helped. To stop relying on psychiatry to 'cure' me; I had to do most of the work.

So Recovery for me was and is creating. You can't go back to the life you had before, and I don't want to. Remember I was 14 and already had a lifetime of abuse before then. I said to myself: life is a stage. What can I do to make it a show worth watching? What song will my heart perform to? I wanted to help others so when I got back to the UK from my trip to the Grand Canyon, I signed up to do voluntary work with BookAid, an organisation that sends books to the poorer parts of the world; and with Crisis, the homeless charity. I also gave blood. I began to feel good about myself. I saw in life something more beautiful than TV watching, anger and hate, which of course meant forgiving my father. That was the hardest thing to do. I wanted to hold onto the pain; I thought it made me what I am. I saw if I didn't forgive him, I was in effect handcuffing myself to the pain for life. Letting go is an amazing feeling. But I am not complacent. There is still much pain to deal with, there are still tears, and there is still anger. I know I haven't forgiven my father 100%, but even 80% will improve your life one thousand fold. As I've got older and made my own mistakes, I saw I had no right to judge my parents. As The Smith's song goes: '[They] are human and need to be loved...'

I think it's fair to say those who have had long-term mental health problems and then have a period of lucidity present itself, realise there are so many things they have missed out on. Moving from insanity to being well is moving from one world to another, and is pretty scary. I mean, what are you supposed to do with your life once you've stopped battling demons? It's very strange being sane and having the memories of a mad person. It is very much like a dreamlike state, and sometimes sanity touches my head like a razorblade pillow.

I tried to make sure my soul and my heart shaped my life and not the habitual responses my early life produced. I pushed myself and challenged myself. I saw giving into fear turn every moment of your soul into a cesspool. You stagnate if you don't reach beyond your fears. I bought a diary and made sure it was filled with good experiences. All the things I was scared to do, I just got up and did. The secret is not to think about it but just get up and do it. Having psychosis makes the road harder, but there is no such thing as impossible.

So one day I just got up and bought a bike - the so longed for bike from childhood. It took me a good few weeks before I got my balance. Suddenly I soared down the street outside my house without falling. 'Weeeeeeeee!' I squealed. I just couldn't stop laughing – and I couldn't stop crying. Tears were streaming down my face. One of my dreams came true. There was no turning back, I had to go forward. I really did have to go forward because I didn't teach myself the brakes on the bike so therefore I *couldn't* stop!

Each of these moments have helped my recovery, but there were moments when I slid back, times of intense pain. No one can escape pain. Nor can anyone escape the ability to learn from the pain. I am still growing. I still believe in my own light. Always believe there is light at the end of the tunnel. There has to be because you are the light. Even when you want to shut down that light and everything seems dark, something shines. It might be a tiny spark buried in an eternity of darkness, but the spark is still there to be seen, it can't be hidden. It is not in its job description to be hidden.

The following things helped my light when it was in danger of dipping.

My parents taught me to handle my emotions badly, and I was always angry at them for this. But this is one more negative emotion to add to the pile they gave me. I decided to go further in my life than my parents: to do more, see more, LIVE more than my parents. I took away power from them back to myself, where it should be.

Fear will be a big part of the journey. There is fear in tackling the past, or creating a new future. Fear is simply believing you aren't strong enough to handle what life brings you, or your issues. You are strong enough. Your amazing strength will blow you away, believe me.

I said to myself: If you live in fear, all those dreams you had will go unaccounted for.

What is it? Most of us live in constant fear, and only a small proportion of our dreams are fulfilled. As a human being we have so much potential, so much that cries out to be done, and when we don't do it, we practice at being dead when we should be alive, and our heart loses it beautiful power. No, I can't submit to fear or not living my dreams, I do not like what I will be otherwise.

I give myself permission to make mistakes, I just don't give myself permission not to learn from my mistakes.

Another thing I tell myself: 'Are you merely a conditioned thing, and not a soul? Are you saying that your conditioning by bad parenting is the way you are going to stay? Do you want to be stuck there?' I thought I would be stuck in that mode. I didn't believe I had the courage to move forward. The thought of it wracked me with fear to step into the unknown. But I so much wanted to move forward that I did challenge my conditioning. Whenever I make a step forward in emotional development, I feel freer, I feel the Dollyness of being Dolly, not what the world around me has shaped me into.

Positivity

You have to act on what you believe. If your mind is focusing on what's missing, you're mind is on what's missing. You are just seeing the hole. Never use a negative ruler to measure your life, it can only measure holes, you can't use it to quantify any good in your life.

Being positive is not denying or being naïve about your shortcomings, it is understanding there is no point lingering in and punishing yourself for those shortcomings. It is asking what can I do to learn from this, what can I do to go beyond this stuckness?

Being positive is not saying all is good, that there are no problems in your life or in the world. Positivity is accepting that there are problems, but being more interested in the solution and be more focussed on that part of it.

Goals

You need them. They don't have to be material goals, it could be spiritual development or to do with your emotions. KNOW YOUR GOAL. BELIEVE YOU CAN REACH YOUR GOAL. ACT ON YOUR BELIEF AND THE STEPS NEEDED TO REACH THE GOAL. AND STAY COMMITTED TO IT. It helps to write your goals down. Things started to change for me when I started committing to goals. For example, I felt lonely and isolated, so I created the goal of going out to social events arranged by local mental health groups. Things like that helped develop my confidence and conversational skills. It was a small goal but had huge repercussions, in that I met Jason Pegler, my publisher at one of these events.

HAVE POSITIVE GOALS, not negative ones. I don't know why, but the brain responds better to positive suggestions rather than negative ones. For example, say: 'I want to have better confidence.' Not: 'I don't want to be lacking in confidence.'

BREAK DOWN YOUR STEPS TO YOUR GOAL INTO MANAGEABLE CHUNKS so you don't feel overwhelmed and disheartened if things don't immediately go your way.

This is a simple formula but hard to do, but all it takes is practice, and you will see changes within months.

There is no magic wand. Somebody said, whether you think you can do something, or think you can't, you're right.

If you think you can do something, then you can.

If you think you can't do something, then you can't.

Simple. But hard to do. But not impossible.

What were the significant points in my life that helped to propel it forward?

1. The decision to change my life for the better and to think more positively.
2. The decision to not to stay at home so much but to interact with more people, which I did by going to a mental health coffee morning run by service users.
3. Travelling to the USA and standing on the Grand Canyon. Its beauty and immensity shamed my negativity and showed me life was worth living.
4. Learning and practicing relaxation techniques. This is where my recovery began. Only a few months of yoga and meditation and everyone, and I mean everyone, noticed the difference.
5. Doing voluntary work: this helped me feel less isolated and that I was contributing to the world and adding light.
6. The continual process of writing; this gave my life meaning and precious content.
7. Number 6 and number 2 merged and I met my publisher Jason Pegler at the aforementioned coffee morning. He was the first person to truly believe in me. This was so empowering, and one of the major changing points in my life. Also, after the publication of the book, opportunity

after opportunity presented themselves, which improved my quality of life and did my self-esteem so much good.

8. Joining a service user group, for support and artistic collaboration. This is a stepping stone. This is tricky one because you have sometimes to deal with people's negativity and their sometimes total identification with their mental health issues. If you are one of the people who want to go beyond that identity and be more yourself, you may find resistance from these people. But having said that, being with various service user groups brought some amazing people and experiences into my life.

9. Getting support in getting my father the proper care he needed. It surprises me that some professionals thought I didn't need support in caring for an abusive father whilst struggling with my own mental health issues. I remember one psychiatrist say to me, 'That's not what we are here for.' I thought they were there to improve my mental health. But by saying that, they proved otherwise. This particular psychiatrist also over-medicated me to the point my father could walk all over me without me having the ability to stand up for myself.

10. I had a dream to make films so I took some courses in film-making. This learning of a new skill, creation of art, and meeting of like-minded made me proud of myself and did me the power of good. The living of a dream is such a powerful and enriching experience; you feel your soul get that little much bigger and stronger.

11. Following on from the previous point, my creativity is my bedrock, my reason for living, the substance of my ambition and dreams, so being able to be creative has always been good to me.

12. I began my public speaking career, mostly speaking to other service users. Making human connection and inspiring people is such an amazing experience. Even if you only do this once in your life, you have made the world that little much better. The light gets bigger.

13. Work: I have to admit to being a workaholic. Maybe this is because I feel I have to catch up after many years lost to psychosis and depression. I realize life is short and I want to leave a legacy to say: Dolly Sen was here. The structure of work also gives structure to my life. My work is my best friend; it is always there to give me strength and meaning and inspiration.

14. Having role models and reading inspirational stories have also been powerful. You realize you don't have to re-invent the wheel. There are people who been there before you who can inspire you with the proof that recovery is very, very possible, and you are not alone. If another human being has done it, than you can do it.

15. Along the same lines as the previous point, finding ways to educate myself about self-improvement, recovery, and positivity.
16. My Buddhism is very valuable to me. Life without spirituality seems empty to me, so it gives me sustenance and inspiration. It also provided me with practical ways to get better. I learnt the very important lesson of having compassion for the self from Buddhism; this is a powerful way to counteract self-hate. Also, through Buddhism, I learnt how to forgive my father, which freed me from him, actually.
17. I mustn't forget my dogs. They give me unconditional love. That is always a good thing!
18. Friends are very important. Family is important. What is the point of life without love? Finding friends is tricky if you are a service user, but it can be done through avenues such as voluntary work, going to college, community projects, mental health social projects and events. It took me a long time to have friends in my life. There was a period of 10 years where I didn't have a single one, but did it through small steps towards a goal.
19. Medication: I have a love/hate relationship with it. Even if the most effective medication is found, the side effects can be horrendous. Sometimes it is nicer to be psychotically high than sedated to the point of sleep, overweight, and with a tremor. The mental health professional has to consider what the person sometimes loses if they take medication. Some people prefer to think they are special in being Jesus, for example, than a drooling sleepwalker. You can lose your symptoms - that is true. But in taking meds, you can lose your quality of life too. But there is no doubting meds help a lot of people regain their quality of life. Good for some people, not so good for others. I am on quite a low dose, and to be honest, it is helping. But the hope is to come off them eventually.
20. Education: being aware of what treatments for psychosis were around and where I could get information about things like housing, social networking, training, complementary therapies, etc.
21. Challenging stigma and discrimination. This is about empowering the powerless. Sometimes stigma and discrimination can be more painful, more paranoia-inducing than psychosis, and need to be challenged. To believe you can advocate on your own behalf empowers the self and improves the lot of others going through similar situations. That is why I do a lot of media work: to educate the wider public and to tell others there is nothing to be ashamed in having mental health issues.
22. Cognitive behaviour therapy (CBT): A lot of the preceding points helped me move along the road to recovery but it was CBT that zoomed

me along that road. Basically, in a nutshell, here I found the tools to control my symptoms, rather than have them control me.

23. Out of the CBT came my rejection of self-pity and the decision to take **total** responsibility for my condition and recovery, and not to expect other to 'cure' me, or wait for others to change so I could change. I had to do the work.

24. Going to university is a dream come true. It gives me a sense of achievement.

25. Learning to laugh at myself. Being human is an absurd and ridiculous career.

26. In all the previous points, there were goals to aim for. I think this is very important. This helps you being pulled towards the future rather the past dictate your path. And to pace yourself with small steps, but the dreams can be as big as you want!

27. And hope. Always have hope. All the previous points have fed the hope I am feeling in the present to make myself a wonderful future.

Like Deegan says, it is the journey of the heart, it is to where the heart can beat its loudest, grow its widest, fly its highest. The heart with your name on it, the only word to the song that wants to be sung out loud.

What I know about recovery?

That it is possible because I am human. And if I see that humanity also in a mental health professional, I will listen to that professional, because we are now connected. Recovery is an ongoing journey, I don't know where it will take me, but I am becoming more and more me. What I know about recovery is that the more you will believe it is possible, the more you will recover. Greatness is not a delusion of grandeur: it is your right. Whether it is being a mum, a writer, a gardener, or helping others. UNIQUENESS – it is yours, isn't it?

II

Two Psychiatrists Look In

Duncan Harding and Frank Holloway

It is a privilege and a pleasure to contribute to this multi-faceted book. This chapter is written by two psychiatrists at different stages in their careers, with an interest in and sympathy towards the principles and practices associated with the term Recovery[1]. Noting Gordon's commitment to Marxism-Leninism, which, although we do not share, we acknowledge the importance of theory. Accordingly we begin by explaining and exploring the differences between nomothetic and idiographic approaches to knowledge, and reflect briefly on the significance of this crucial distinction to the reception of Recovery in an academic and professional context. We explore what the term Recovery means to mental health care professionals in today's NHS. We discuss ways in which Recovery may be evaluated and measured, and the relevance of outcome measures. We attempt to deconstruct the concept of Recovery, and consider some of the main criticisms of the term and its meaning. We then go on to consider potential pathways to Recovery, in terms of both service provision and also on a more personal level. Finally, we reflect on Gordon's story, and on what lessons might be learned that could have more widespread implications for the design and modelling of recovery-based mental health services. As psychiatrists we perforce use terms, such as 'patient' 'illness' and 'disability', which others might have difficulty with: these terms are both descriptive and identify the conceptual framework within which we work.

The 'nomothetic' and the 'idiographic'

The terms *'nomothetic'* and its opposite *'idiographic'* were coined by the now obscure 19th Century philosopher Wilhelm Windelband to describe two distinct approaches to knowledge which are neatly defined in *Wikipedia*. (http://en.wikipedia.org/wiki/Nomothetic_and_idiographic Accessed 27/12/08).

---

1. Recovery is throughout this chapter capitalised and italicised to emphasise the complexity and ambiguity of the term with some specific exceptions, where it is being used in its ordinary-language meaning.

The *nomothetic* is based on what Immanuel Kant described as a tendency to generalize, and is typically expressed in the natural sciences. It involves the effort to derive general laws relating to objectively determined phenomena. Physics, chemistry, cosmology and molecular genetics are clearly based on the *nomothetic* approach to knowledge. Psychiatrists obtain their qualifications by passing examinations that require a good grasp of natural sciences and many progress in their careers by contributing to the evidence-base for psychiatric practice using methodologies derived from the natural sciences. Evidence-based medicine, which mental health practitioners are required to undertake, is a *nomothetic*, rule bound activity.

The *idiographic* is based on what Kant described as a tendency to specify, and is typically expressed in the humanities. It describes the effort to understand the meaning of contingent, accidental, and often subjective phenomena. Nomothetic approaches to understanding tend to be quantitative, statistical and population-based. Idiographic approaches, in contrast, relate to the study of an individual, who is seen as an entity, with properties setting him/her apart from other individuals and are in general qualitative. (Some attempts have been made to develop quantitative idiographic research methods in psychology, for example Shapiro's Personal Questionnaire). When we experience ill-health personally this is inevitably understood in personal, narrative terms and the mental health literature is increasingly the richer for such first-person accounts. Everyone working effectively within mental health services requires a profound interest in the individual, their unique personal history and social context.

The nomothetic/idiographic distinction has been particularly important in understanding work in psychology, sociology and anthropology, where there is clear and obvious tension between population-based, statistical approaches and those that try and identify individual personal meanings. It is also highly relevant to understanding the complexities surrounding the current discourse on *Recovery* within mental health services, which can be quite legitimately understood in both nomothetic and idiographic terms.

To put this crudely *Recovery* can be conceptualised in nomothetic terms: the 'objectively' measured outcomes for populations of individuals with particular characteristics (specific 'mental illnesses') and the 'evidence-based' service inputs that 'optimise' these outcomes. This is often seen as a reductionistic and rather inhumane way of addressing human distress. Equally we can seek to understand *Recovery* in an idiographic framework that is captured in the individual narratives of people experiencing extreme mental distress and, in their own particular way, transcending that distress. These narratives might then inform others experiencing their own individual journey through distress and people who would seek to help them. The idiographic approach can seem naïve and anecdotal but is also capable of being extremely sophisticated (see for example Davidson, 2003 who uses phenomenological analysis to make sense of individual experience of recovery in schizophrenia).

There can of course also be leakage between the nomothetic and idiographic word views. Thus an idiographic study can be carried out obtaining very rich narratives from people living with schizophrenia – itself a profoundly nomothetic concept. Conversely the narratives of people about the nature of their life stories and what has helped and hindered them – idiographic material – can be important in sparking off a line of research that increases the nomothetic evidence base.

As we can see the same word, 'recovery', is regularly used to look at mental illness or mental distress from two entirely different intellectual perspectives. In general, individuals using the term do not describe (or perhaps even fully grasp) the conceptual framework(s) within which they are working. Little wonder that although the *Recovery* paradigm is dominant within mental health policy in the United Kingdom (CSIP, 2007; Shepherd et al, 2008), Ireland and indeed throughout the English-speaking world (Ramon et al, 2007) people – staff, service users and academic commentators - don't necessarily know what they disagree with or are required to be signed up to.

Understanding Recovery: The doctors' dilemma

Jerome Carson (Chapter 7, this book) summarises the vast literature on *Recovery*. Two broad ways of understanding the concept are usually identified (Resnick *et al*, 2004). These might loosely be characterised as (1) the ordinary-language *nomothetic* concept of 'recovery-as-getting-better' and (2) the contemporary *idiographic* conceptualisation of 'recovery as a journey of the heart', a deeply individual process that is linked with finding personal meaning even in the face of ongoing illness and disability (Deegan, 1996). However a third strand can be found within the recovery literature (Holloway, 2008). This focuses on the rights of people living with mental illness to social inclusion and self-determination and springs from the broader disability rights movement (Davidson *et al*, 2006).

From the medical perspective to understand recovery we must first understand what the person is recovering from. Take for example the ophthalmologist. A person may present to the doctor with near blindness.

Following a relatively fast and pain free cataract operation under local anaesthetic the person may regain near perfect sight. With regards to the person's vision they have indeed recovered in the ordinary sense of the term. This outcome for treatment of cataract is expected and usual and from the first meeting the doctor and patient have a shared mutual feeling of hope and optimism: the transaction between doctor and patient is a relatively simple one.

The psychiatrist, particularly one working in a rehabilitation or long-term care setting, is often working with a person experiencing a chronic and pervasive illness that affects many aspects of their life and well-being. Psychiatrists are trained to think in terms of symptoms and diagnoses, illness, disability and impairment in social functioning. This language fits rather badly with the rhetoric associated with *Recovery*. However the psychiatrist will (or certainly should) be interested in the person as a whole, and will require a holistic view of what recovery means to that person that goes beyond merely addressing the presenting symptomatology. Whilst there are many examples of people returning to a normal level of function after treatment of a psychiatric illness, the psychiatrist will also see people who may never again experience their prior levels of functioning. Here the transaction between doctor and patient becomes much more complex.

In fact much of medical practice involves similarly complex interactions: even the ophthalmologist will be spending a great deal of time working with people whose conditions are degenerative or irreversible. In such cases the patient may lose their sight but by no means does that imply that they cannot live a good life, transcending the apparent catastrophe of blindness (although in that particular case the doctor's role in helping the person to live a good life will be distinctly limited).

The first-person literature attests that *Recovery* starts with a person finding hope – hope that is so easily eroded and washed away if mental health professionals do not nurture a person's optimism for the future with every interaction. (Professionals might argue that alongside this may be the need to help a person attain a realistic impression of what they might hope for and setting the goal-posts of recovery depending on their particular illness, although such an attitude may be seen as unnecessarily limiting and paternalistic). One effect of severe mental disorder is for people to lose their sense of self. *Recovery* may involve a person rediscovering their identity and finding meaning in their life (Davidson and Strauss, 1992). Social exclusion is an almost universal consequence of severe mental disorder: *Recovery* will be leading towards social inclusion and allowing people to reconnect with and to stamp their mark on society. Mental disorder and the ways society manage it frequently result in a loss of a person's autonomy (quite dramatically when people are forced into hospital and compelled to take treatments they may not want, but equally and more pervasively in multiple undramatic ways). In these circumstances *Recovery* may involve a person regaining their autonomy and taking responsibility for their future.

The dilemma for doctors, and indeed other health care professionals, is to find a middle way that allows us to retain an objective perspective on our understanding of the nature of the problems people are presenting with that attention to individual meanings that the *idiographic Recovery* literature emphasises. 'Values-based' practice is promoted as a toolkit for practitioners to balance the conflicting values people (society, patients, carers and professionals) bring to health care in the same way that 'evidence-based' practice seeks to ensure that professionals make the best decisions in the face of a confusing and conflicting evidence base (see for example Fulford 2004). (See the Warwick Medical School website on values-based practice for an accessible brief introduction, http://www2.warwick.ac.uk/fac/med/study/cpd/subject_index/pemh/vbp_introduction.)

In principle it may be a way of bridging the conceptual gap between the professional and lay world views of mental illness.

The implications of *Recovery* for practitioners

It follows from the *idiographic* approach to *Recovery* that as health care professionals we must enable a person to have as much choice as possible, allowing them to guide their own *Recovery*. As we understand it *Recovery* is enabled by a transfer of power back to the patient, who should of course be given all the benefits that healthcare can offer but in a manner that is experienced as empowering in order to give them the tools to fashion their own *Recovery*. The power should not be in the hands of the doctor or other practitioner: it should be squarely with the patient. This can be achieved partly through a collaborative approach to treatment.

Recovery is not necessarily about a person once again going about life as they used to before – sometimes it is about a person accepting the long-term nature of their illness, and despite any limitations this causes finding hope and meaning in their life. (Alternatively, of course, it may be that something about a person's life as it was lived before the onset of the illness contributed to the illness, necessitating a change in lifestyle or approach to life.). If hope is an important ingredient in personal *Recovery* – as people's narratives tell us it is – then practitioners need to find ways of instilling hope even in the face of continuing symptomatology and disability. Similarly health care professionals and peer supporters need to learn ways of helping people re-establish their own identity, find their place in the world and find meaning in their life.

In the research driven world of evidence-based medical practice it is often easy to forget the individual stories of hope and recovery that in themselves may guide our practice of medicine. We are trained to critically assess literature with regards to the quality of research design, statistical power and authenticity. As we have seen, medical practice is necessarily informed by *nomothetic* discourse that deals in knowledge acquired through natural-scientific methodologies. However, it has become increasingly recognised that one person's *idiographic* story can be just as powerful and informative as a large multi-centre clinical trial, if that story leads to a doctor re-assessing his or her clinical practice and incorporating the lessons learnt into other people's care. As doctors working in mental health services we have learned invaluable lessons from the personal stories of recovery and rehabilitation that we have had the privilege to witness first hand. Each one of these stories is unique, and has helped to shape our understanding of *Recovery* and our practice as psychiatrists. Gordon's story is a good example of this, and having read this book so far you will no doubt appreciate the potential of his personal story of recovery to shape future practice.

Measuring *Recovery*

Health professionals and researchers understand recovery in terms of a range of outcomes that can be objectively, or perhaps more accurately, reliably and validly, assessed. Reliability is the extent to which measurement would be the same if undertaken again or by someone else. Validity is the extent to which the measure captures what it is supposed to. Thus the ophthalmologist will assess visual acuity after a cataract operation – a measure that maps fairly well onto the real-world experience of the patient as far as recovery of eyesight is concerned. (More subtly and skilfully the ophthalmologist may be assessing the state of the fundus –that is the back of the eye – of someone with diabetes following laser treatment designed to correct lesions in the blood vessels that would threaten sight without the patient having any awareness of the potentially sight-endangering problems they had been experiencing.)

Within mental health services research a very wide range of outcome measures can be used. These cover the domains of experience that are known to be affected by mental illness/mental disorder as well as measures that may be of more concern to the policy-maker than the patient (such as service use and cost). The Table (first column) lists commonly-used domains of outcome measures in the research literature. Psychiatrists focus particularly on symptoms, and it is therefore no surprise that there are multiple outcome measures available that measure the symptoms that people are experiencing with admirable reliability. There are tools with demonstrated reliability and validity available that can be used to assess outcomes in all these 'nomothetic' areas: none is without difficulties and researchers have to be careful in selecting the right measure for the particular issue being studied. Working within this tradition Liberman and Kopelowicz (2005) put forward an operational definition of recovery from schizophrenia. This requires low levels of symptomatology using the Brief Psychiatric Rating Scale (Ventura et al, 1993) and the person demonstrating aspects of social functioning (in terms of occupation, self-management and social interaction), both sustained over a period of time. In the absence of a clear definition of what is meant by recovery scientists cannot communicate with each other.

Table 1
Recovery outcome measurement: 'Nomothetic' vs. 'Idiographic' outcomes

Nomothetic outcomes	Idiographic outcomes
Data	Narrative
Symptom reduction	Empowerment
Improved social functioning	Hope
Decreased social disability	Healing
Improved subjective quality of life	Sense of self
Increased social inclusion:	Connection
Housing	
Employment	
Social networks	
Intimate relationships	
Decreased use of services	
No hospital admissions	
Reduction in inpatient bed days	
Discharge from services	
Service-related costs	
Decreased offending behaviour	

Historically outcome measures have been much less regularly deployed in routine clinical practice. In England, as part of the Mental Health Minimum Dataset, clinicians are supposed to be assessing their clients/patients regularly using the Health of the Nation Outcomes Scales (HoNOS) (Wing et al, 1996). HoNOS seeks to measure both symptoms and social functioning and one of the authors (FH) now receives regular feedback on the outcomes recorded for his patients using HoNOS.

Changes in HoNOS scores are opaque representations of a person's experience. Those working within the *idiographic* tradition would argue that more important is how a person measures and evaluates their own recovery. There are many personal accounts of recovery and learning to live with illness that have been key in driving recovery principles in modern medical practice (e.g. Chamberlin, 1978; Deegan, 1988, 1996; Clay, 1994; Ridgeway, 2000). It has been argued that focussing on the individual perspectives of those recovering from mental illness helps to fight stigma (Leibrich, 1999; Ramsay et al., 2002). These narratives emphasise the importance of hope, empowerment, connectedness, healing and sense of self (see Table, second column)

In fact long-term outcome studies support a more hopeful and optimistic attitude towards *Recovery* in the *nomothetic* sense than is often believed. Because professionals only see people with continuing problems they tend to perceive the outcomes for severe mental illness as rather worse than they actually are. (For examples of outcome studies in schizophrenia see the very long term studies by Harding *et al.*, 1987 and Harrison et al, 2001 and partial reviews of the literature in Warner, 1994; Liberman and Kopelowicsz, 2005; and Ramon et al, 2007). The outcome literature can be criticised for its excessive focus on symptoms and disability at the expense of investigating 'recovering a meaningful and fulfilling life within the limitations of the disorder' (Harrison *et al.*, 2001).

Finding meaning in life, even in the face of chronic disability, is a key element of *Recovery*. This is a personal and unique experience that is not necessarily readily tabulated and easily presented in a scientific paper. Indeed, trying to generalise these personal narratives and experiences may in itself detract from the strength of the individual perspective. It is, however, possible to extract core features and themes that underlie recovery narratives that one could use to inform current practice.

In an age of evidence-based medical practice, when the results of countless interventions have been measured meticulously for over a century, collated and used to drive further developments in practice, meaningful outcome measures that tap into the person-centred conceptualisation of *Recovery* are still in their infancy (Roberts & Wolfson, 2004). Also in their infancy are measures that look at the extent to which a service might and does promote *Recovery* for its users. There is very limited experience with currently available tools, such as the DREEM (Dinniss et al , 2007).

Deconstructing Recovery

It has been argued that the concept of *Recovery* has the potential to fundamentally change mental health theory and practice (Ramon *et al.*, 2007). However, it is important to remember that the concept needs to be carefully and critically analysed and its meaning clarified, as well as the implications it has at all levels from service users to Government policy (Ramon *et al.*, 2007).

Recovery is not without its critics. It is generally considered to be a personal process unique to each recovering person. Its definition in the literature reflects this in allowing individualised flexibility (Ramon *et al.*, 2007). However, since *Recovery* is not sharply defined it is sometimes felt that the concept lacks any meaning at all. A further concern is that *Recovery* could be seen as a way to further shift responsibility away from society and services to the individual service user (Ramon *et al.*, 2007). It has been proposed that de-institutionalisation only became socially acceptable once it was perceived that people with mental illness could be effectively cared for and regulated in the community (Scull, 1977). *Recovery* could be seen as one more step to absolve society and the state of responsibility to those who are mentally ill. *Recovery* could therefore be cynically viewed as a way of absolving responsibility and saving money. The person centred focus of the movement perhaps make this unlikely, particularly since Government has taken the core tenets of *Recovery* to the heart of mental health policy in England (Department of Health, 2001). The current health and social care policy agenda heavily emphasises the importance of self-directed care and personalisation in the management of long-term conditions.

Recovery can also be seen as either 'old news' or a 'fad'. Some people will argue that 'we had been doing recovery anyway' and others that *Recovery* is the latest 'flavour of the month' that 'sets people up for failure' (Davidson *et al.*, 2006). Critics of *Recovery* may also say that recovery-oriented care adds further burden to already stretched health care professionals, and that it increases the service provider's exposure to risk and liability (Davidson *et al.*, 2006). Even as it stands without any extra burden of activity, despite an ethical imperative to promote the autonomy of the patient/service user, many practitioners would acknowledge that in reality one can sometimes get caught up in the chaos of a busy job. Too often the underlying principle of patient care becomes what will get us through the day. There is a danger of an institutionalised gap occurring between the rhetoric of *Recovery*-oriented practice and reality.

Promoting *Recovery*

Practitioners of rehabilitation psychiatry typically work with people who are identified as having 'failed' within the mainstream service system by dint of 'treatment resistance', lengthy hospital admission and severe social disability. They regularly experience that good outcomes occur when people suffering from an illness deemed 'refractory' are treated with respect and dignity and are nursed back to health in a therapeutic setting that is optimistic and encourages mutual collaboration (Craig, 2006). There is nothing new about this insight: the spectacularly successful deinstitutionalisation movement that closed most of our mental hospitals was based on similar principles, albeit expressed in the rather different terminologies of social therapy, social psychiatry and latterly normalisation (Clark, 1974; Wolfensberger 1983). As a corollary we have long known quite a bit about practices that lead to institutionalisation and disempowerment (Wing and Brown, 1970).

For *Recovery* to be achieved on an individual level psychiatric practice must offer an environment that encourages and nurtures it. Doctors and other mental health professionals need to work alongside the patient in a collaboration that aims for the common goal of *Recovery*. The professional provides expert knowledge and skills in diagnosis and then arms the patient with the building blocks required to achieve their individual *Recovery* goals. The professional must allow the patient as much autonomy and choice as possible with regards to treatment options and in return the patient must take responsibility for the treatment choices they make. In this paradigm the professional shifts their role from an authority in the field to that of a coach or personal trainer (Roberts & Wolfson, 2004). The professional provides expert knowledge that has been previously gathered regarding a particular illness and the patient provides expert knowledge of their own illness. The patient is an 'expert by experience' (Roberts & Wolfson, 2004).

Everyone is influenced by those around them. The experiences of a person enduring distressing and disorienting experiences is influenced by the attitude of the psychiatrist and other mental health professionals they encounter on their journey as a patient. A patient must feel from the very first interaction with the mental health professional that they are working alongside someone who really believes in them as a person, and who has hope for their future.

However there are important nuances here. Whilst it may be important to impress the seriousness of a given situation (for example to explain why compulsory detention in hospital has been instituted or educate and facilitate compliance with medication) the mental health professional must always strike a balance between acceptance and hope. It may be the case that acceptance of illness comes hand in hand with hope for the future. It is often the case that the patient has been suffering with distressing symptoms, or unpleasant consequences of their actions whilst unwell. Accepting the reality of their illness and agreeing to treatment can give clarity to their situation and will allow the possibility of hope for the future, as well as relief from distressing symptoms.

Professionals give careful thought to the timing of fully explaining the details and implications of an illness to a patient matched to the patient's ability and desire to accept these explanations (McGorry, 1992). Just as a person goes through natural phases of bereavement, a patient may be in a period of denial with regards to their illness, and this denial may in fact be helpful in itself (Deegan, 1988). A patient should not be stripped of denial too early, and some commentators advocate 'avoid(ing) adding insight to injury' (McGorry 1992). It should also be appreciated that if a person sees significance in the presence of particular symptoms (e.g. psychotic symptoms) then they will likely see significance in their absence also: consequently the losses experienced by a recovering patient are extremely complex (Roberts, 2000). This complex and dynamic pattern of resistance needs to be carefully considered in *Recovery*, and there is growing evidence to suggest that it may be more helpful to work with psychotic symptoms rather than expending all efforts to prove them false (Roberts & Wolfson, 2004).

With regards to treatment options and medication, the psychiatrist is increasingly operating more like their medical and surgical colleagues who provide an expert diagnosis and then give a variety of management options for the patient to choose from (Davidson *et al.*, 2006). Legally defined decision-making capacity is often impaired during acute exacerbations of mental illness (and may be lacking when the illness is prolonged) (Owen et al, 2008). When a patient lacks the capacity to give consent for a particular treatment, they must be given as much choice and autonomy as possible. There are usually different options with regards to medication, and the patient should be involved as much as possible in that decision making process. If a patient is too unwell to make a choice then a decision should be made in their best interests, but they should be consulted and involved in treatment decisions at the earliest opportunity. In this way a patient is given autonomy, and with autonomy comes responsibility - responsibility for their own treatment choices and ultimately for their own *Recovery*.

Beyond the doctor-patient interaction, there are other practical and conceptual aspects of mental health services that need to be optimised to facilitate recovery (Davidson, 2005). Social inclusion is key to achieving *Recovery*, and the main obstacles for this experienced by service users are social deprivation and disadvantage (ODPM, 2004). Mental health services have been restructured to meet the needs of people in the form of new community teams dealing with crisis resolution, assertive outreach, and early intervention. Within teams there is an increased emphasis on a patient centred/recovery approach (for example, employing Support, Time and Recovery workers). Some people have noted a shift in the concept of the nature of the symptoms of mental illness, with a move away from the idea that the symptoms represent an illness and towards the concept that these experiences are a shared human process. There is also a move towards a person being 'the architect of one's own recovery'. This implies a more individual approach, rather than a person being a 'recipient patient' who is fitted into a collective solution aiming for recovery (Davidson, 2005). Authorities emphasise the importance of peer-led services in promoting *Recovery*, something that is much more common in the United States than the United Kingdom (Davidson et al, 2006).

On a more personal and psychological level, it has been proposed that there are four main conceptual components of psychological recovery: finding hope; finding one's self identity; finding meaning in one's life; and taking responsibility for one's own recovery (Andresen *et al.*, 2003). Stages of recovery have been identified by several studies (Davidson & Strauss, 1992; Baxter & Diehl, 1998; Pettie & Triolo, 1999; Young & Ensing, 1999; Spaniol *et al.*, 2002). These stages can be summarised in the following five steps. Firstly there is a stage of moratorium, characterised by denial, confusion and hopelessness, leading to the second stage of awareness, when the person first experiences hope and realises they are capable of recovery (Andresen *et al.*, 2003). The third stage is that of preparation, when the person assesses one's strengths and weaknesses, and also becomes educated as to the help and services that are available to them. This leads onto the crucial stage of rebuilding, when the person rebuilds their identity and takes responsibility for their treatment and recovery. The final stage is that of growth – this is the outcome of the recovery process, and during this stage the person manages their own illness, though not necessarily symptom free, and also is resilient in the face of ongoing illness and maintains a positive outlook to live a full and meaningful life (Andresen *et al.*, 2003). A strikingly similar formulation is to be found in the *Recovery Star*, a *Recovery*-oriented outcome measure that has recently been developed in the UK. Here the five stages, which are assessed in ten life domains, move from 'stuck', through 'accessing help', 'believing' (that change is possible) and 'learning' (how to change) to ''self-reliance' (McKeith and Burns, 2008).

Conclusions

In reality *Recovery* is not a particularly new concept. Its major tenets were seen in the move towards 'moral treatment' of the early 19th Century and concerns that emerged in the mid 19th Century about the welfare of people consigned to life in an asylum. The key issues relevant to *Recovery* re-emerged within Social Psychiatry in the 1960s and 1970s and during the process of de-institutionalisation in the 1980s and 1990s. *Recovery* also borrows significantly from the Disability Rights movement that has been so successful in recent decades.

In essence *Recovery* is about a person-centred approach to psychiatric care and rehabilitation. It will be facilitated by changes in all levels of care, from government policy to a doctor's language and attitude. *Recovery* is about instilling hope and enabling a person to find meaning in their life. It is about an environment that promotes social inclusion and allows a person with a mental health problem to take control of their life. *Recovery* is about empowerment, and shifting power from a doctor or other mental health professional to the patient. *Recovery* is about collaboration between professional and patient. Ultimately, *Recovery* is about working together to aim towards the patient experiencing a good life, whatever the nature of their symptomatology or disability. However patients and professionals must acknowledge that there are circumstances when collaboration breaks down and (legally sanctioned) compulsion supervenes or when professionals are taking decisions for people who lack decision-making capacity. These actions need to be understood by all participants and with good will should not undermine the individual's *Recovery* journey.

Gordon's story is unique, as are all narratives of personal paths to recovery. As we have discussed, growth in the understanding of *Recovery* is largely driven by personal narrative and service user's own experiences and stories.

References

Andresen, R., Oades, L. and Caputi , P. (2003) The experience of recovery from schizophrenia: towards an empirically validated state model. *Australian and New Zealand Journal of Psychiatry*; **37**: 586-594.

Baxter, E. A. and Diehl, S. (1998) Emotional Stages: Consumers and family members recovering from the trauma of mental illness. *Psychiatric Rehabilitation Journal*; **22**: 186-188.

Care Services Improvement Partnership (2007) *A common purpose: Recovery in future mental health services Joint Position Paper 08* Leeds: CSIP.

Chamberlin, J. (1978) *On Our Own: patient controlled alternatives to the mental health system*. New York: McGraw-Hill.

Clark, D.H. (1974) *Social Therapy in Psychiatry*. Harmonsdworth: Penguin.

Clay, S. (1994) The wounded prophet. In *Recovery: The New Force in Mental Health*. Columbus OH: Ohio Department of Mental Health.

Craig, T. (2006) What is psychiatric rehabilitation? In Roberts, G. Davenport, S. Holloway, F. & Tattan, T. (Eds) *Enabling Recovery: The Principles and Practice of Rehabilitation Psychiatry*. London: Gaskell.

Davidson L (2003) *Living Outside Mental Illness. Qualitative Studies on Recovery in Schizophrenia*. New York: New York University Press.

Davidson, L. (2005) Recovery, Self Management and the Expert Patient. *Journal of Mental Health*; **14** (1): 25-35.

Davidson, L., O'Connell, M., Tondora, J., Styron, T. and Kangas, K. (2006) The top ten concerns about recovery encountered in mental health service transformation. *Psychiatric Services*; **57** (5): 640-645.

Davidson, L. and Strauss, J. (1992) Sense of self in recovery from severe mental illness. *British Journal of Medical Psychology* ; **65**: 131-145.

Deegan, P. E. (1988) Recovery: the lived experience of rehabilitation. *Psychosocial Rehabilitation Journal*; **11**: 136-138.

Deegan, P. (1996) Recovery as a journey of the heart. *Psychiatric Rehabilitation Journal*; **19**: 91-97.

Department of Health (2001) *The Journey to Recovery – The Government's Vision for Mental Health Care*. London: Department of Health.

Dinniss S, Roberts G, Hubbard C, Mounsell J and Webb R (2007) User-led assessment of recovery using DREEM. *Psychiatric Bulletin*, 31, 124-127.

Fulford, K.W.M. (2004) Ten Principles of Values-Based Medicine. In Radden, J. (Ed) *The Philosophy of Psychiatry: A Companion*. New York: Oxford University Press.

Harding, C. M., Brooks, G. W., Asolaga, T. S. J. S. and Brier, A. (1987) The Vermont longitudinal study of persons with severe mental illness. 1:

Methodological study sample and overall status 32 years later. *American Journal of Psychiatry*; **144**: 718-726.

Harrison, G. Hopper, K., Craig, T et al. (2001) Recovery from psychotic illness: a 15- and 25-year international follow-up study. *British Journal of Psychiatry*; **178**: 506-517.

Holloway F (2008) Is there a science of recovery and does it matter? Invited Commentary on: Recovery and the Medical Model. *Advances in Psychiatric Treatment*, 14, 245-247

Leibrich, J. (1999) *A Gift of Stories: Discovering How to Deal with Mental Illness.* Dunedin: University of Otago Press.

Liberman RP and Kopelowicz A (2005) Recovery from schizophrenia: a concept in search of research. *Psychiatric Services*, 56, 735-742.

McGorry, P. D. (1992) The concept of recovery and secondary prevention in psychotic disorders. *Australian and New Zealand Journal of Psychiatry*; **26**: 3-17.

MacKieth J and Burns S (2008) *Mental Health Recovery Star.* London: Mental Health Providers Forum.

Office of the Deputy Prime Minister (2004) *Mental Health and Social Exclusion.* London: Office of the Deputy Prime Minister

Owen GS, Richardson G, David A et al (2008) Mental capacity to make decisions on treatment in people admitted to psychiatric hospitals: cross-sectional study. *British Medical Journal*, 337, a448

Pettie, D. and Triolo, A. M. (1999) Illness as evolution: The search for identity and meaning in the recovery process. *Psychiatric Rehabilitation Journal*; **22**: 255-262.

Ramon, S. Healy, B. and Renouf, N. (2007) Recovery from mental illness as an emergent concept and practice in Australia and the UK. *International Journal of Social Psychiatry*; **53**: 108-122.

Ramsay, R., Page, A. Goodman, T., and Hart, G. (2002) Changing Minds: Our Lives and Mental Illness. London: Gaskell.

Resnick, S. Rosenheck, R. and Lehman, A. (2004) An exploratory analysis of correlates of recovery. *Psychiatric Services*, 55, 5, 540-547.

Ridgeway, P. A. (2000) Re-storying psychiatric disability: learning from first person narrative accounts of recovery. *Psychiatric Rehabilitation Journal*; **24**: 335-343.

Roberts, G. A. (2000) Narrative and severe mental illness: what place do stories have in an evidence based world? *Advances in Psychiatric Treatment*; **6**: 432-441.

Roberts, G. and Wolfson, P. (2004) The rediscovery of recovery: open to all. *Advances in Psychiatric Treatment*; **10**: 37-49.

Scull, A. (1977) Decarceration: A Radical View. Englewood Cliffs, NJ: Prentice-Hall.

Shepherd G, Boardman J and Slade M (2008). *Making Recovery a Reality.* London;

Sainsbury Centre for Mental Health.

Spaniol, L., Wewiorski, N., Gagne, C. and Anthony, W. A. (2002) The process of recovery from schizophrenia. *International Review of Psychiatry*; **14**: 327-336.

Ventura, M.A., Green, M.F., Shaner, A. & Liberman, R.P. (1993). Training and quality assurance with the brief psychiatric rating scale: 'The drift buster'. *International Journal of Methods in Psychiatric Research*, 3, 221-244.

Warner, R. (1994) *Recovery from Schizophrenia: Psychiatry and Political Economy (2nd edn)*. New York: Routledge.

Wing, J. K. & Brown, G. W. (1970) *Institutionalism and Schizophrenia: A Comparative Study of Three Mental Hospitals 1960–1968*. Cambridge: Cambridge University Press.

Wing, J., Curtis, R. and Beevor, A. S. (1996) Health of the Nations Outcomes Scales (HoNOS). London: Royal College of Psychiatrists' Research Unit.

Wolfensberger W (1983) Social role valorization: a proposed new term for the principle of normalization. *Mental Retardation*, 21, 234–9.

Young, S. L. and Ensing, D. S. (1999) Exploring recovery from the perspective of people with psychiatric disabilities. *Psychiatric Rehabilitation Journal*; **22**: 219-231.

12

The right to contribute: Employment and recovery

Rachel Perkins

As Rachel states in her introduction, she had been working in mental health services as a psychologist for a decade, before she developed mental health problems herself. As she puts it, she then crossed that dividing line from the sane to the mad. When thinking about when to go back to work after her breakdown, her psychiatrist advised waiting until she was "really ready." Another person suggested that maybe being a psychologist was too stressful. In the end it was the support of 'friends and loved ones, and a boss, who believed in me' that propelled her back to work. Her main passion then and thereafter has been the fight for the right to proper access to real employment opportunities for people with mental health problems. As she points out, 'Unemployment can so easily lead to the loss of all identities other than that of mental patient and reinforces the notion that we have little (if anything) to contribute.' She stresses the importance of hope and hope inspiring relationships, taking back control of your life and the right to have opportunities to contribute. No other mental health professional has done more to highlight the importance of employment in recovery.

Maybe it's because of my Quaker upbringing, or perhaps the revolutionary socialism of my early teens imbued in me a belief in the dignity of labour. Or possibly it is just that, whether we like it or not, we live in a society where our work defines us. It is the second question when you meet someone new: 'What is your name? What do you do? And doing manic depression is a serious conversation stopper. Whatever the reason, my work – as a mental health professional, as a writer, as a campaigner – lies at the core of my identity and my life.

> This is my workplace. This is where I earn my definition, the place that tells me what I am. (Galloway, 1991).

I had been working in mental health services for a decade, before I was formerly diagnosed ... before I added to my two psychiatric careers (as professional and writer/campaigner) a third – as a 'mental patient'. At first getting a diagnosis was something of a relief - kind of liberating. Maybe some of the problems I was having - at work, with people, with meeting commitments - resulted not, as I had supposed, from my utter incompetence and uselessness, but from the fact that something was wrong. Perhaps I could receive the absolution I needed for failing to live up to the expectations (my own and those of others) that I had hitherto taken so easily in my stride (Perkins, 1999).

But the relief that knowing 'something was wrong' was tempered by very real fear. I knew all the statistics about prejudice, discrimination, exclusion. I had seen their consequences in the lives of people with whom I worked. What I could not know, until I faced them myself, was their lived reality and just how desperate and hopeless I would feel. I was astounded at how little my career as a mental health professional equipped me for life on the other side – as a 'mental patient'. I found myself completely at sea not really knowing what to do and feeling very alone. There are no guidelines about how to be a recipient of mental health services. No-one tells you the rules. There were people around trying valiantly to help, but somehow I could not make contact with them as I usually did. An intangible barrier seemed to divide us. I had crossed that 'no-(wo)man's land' that divides 'them' from 'us' - the mad from the sane.

I was convinced that I would lose everything I valued in life: my friends, my home, my sports car and most of all, my job – my hitherto successful career – that underpinned all the things that I held dear. Remember, this was back in the early 1990s before disability rights legislation, in the days when the Clothier 'two year rule' reigned supreme (Clothier, 1994). A rule that said no-one should be employed in the NHS within two years of having received treatment for a mental health condition. I really could be sacked simply because I had a mental health condition.

The messages I received from the mental health professionals helping me did little to dissuade me of the hopelessness of my situation. When I asked my psychiatrist when I could go back to work her undoubtedly well-meaning response was that I should not return until I felt 'really ready'. I am sure she was trying to help assuage my guilt for being 'off sick', but what I heard in her response was 'I don't think you are really ready to go back'. And anyone who has been off work for a period of time for whatever reason knows that the longer you are off, the less ready to go back you feel. It's not rocket science. Even my grandmother knew that if you fell off a bicycle you should get back on as soon as possible. Then there was the, undoubtedly well-meant, advice that maybe being a clinical psychologist was too stressful – maybe I should look for a less demanding job.

I was convinced my life was over ... and I am not alone.

'Out of the blue your job is gone, and with it any financial security you may have had. At a stroke, you have no purpose in life, and no contact with other people. You find yourself totally isolated from the rest of the world. No one telephones you. Much less writes. No-one seems to care if you are alive or dead.' (Bird, 2001)

... I was 19 and had the same ambitions as any other 19 year old. I had hoped to make a place in the world for myself. But instead I was a patient in a hospital ... the vocational rehabilitation counsellor ... said 'Well there's nothing much I have to offer you; I can see from your records that you'll never be capable of holding a job.' Tears came to my eyes; I thought all the facts were in. At the age of 19, when most people are eagerly anticipating and planning for the future, I had been told that I had nothing to look forward to but a 'career' as a ward of the state. (Rogers, 1995)

My job was my life, I felt my life was destroyed. (Bodman et al, 2003)

A right denied?

The right to work is enshrined in Article 23 of the United Nations Declaration of Human Rights (1948),

Everyone has the right to work, to free choice of employment, to just and favourable conditions of work and to protection against unemployment.

Yet this remains a right denied to many people with a mental health condition. Studies repeatedly show that the vast majority of people with a mental health condition would like to work, indeed people with mental health conditions have the highest 'want to work' rate of any disabled people (Social Exclusion Unit, 2004). Few have the opportunity to do so. The overall employment rate stands at around 74%, the employment rate for disabled people in general is 47%, yet the employment rate for people with a mental health condition in 21%. The proportion of people with a mental health condition claiming incapacity benefit has risen from around 30% in 1999 to 43% in 2008 and continues to rise (see Perkins et al, 2009).

I am one of a very lucky few. Despite having a recurring mental health condition that takes me back to a psychiatric ward every couple of years or so, I had the choice to return to work and pursue my career thanks to friends and loved ones, and a boss, who believed in me when I found it hard to believe in myself.

For almost three decades I have been arguing and campaigning for everyone to enjoy the choice I had: the right of people with a mental health condition to work and receive all the support and help they need to do so. I have initiated a range of programmes designed to achieve this (see, for example, Rinaldi & Perkins, 2007; Rinaldi et al, 2004; Perkins et al, 2010).

In the climate of the Thatcher years - when people who were out of work were being encouraged to move to incapacity benefits in an attempt to make the alarmingly high unemployment figures look less bad - it was easy to talk about, and campaign around, the right to work. In 2010 we live in changed economic times when the desire is to reverse this process: reduce the 'rising tide' of incapacity benefits claimants (many of whom appear to be moving from the higher level incapacity benefits to lower level unemployment benefits – often still with no job, but with less money each week to live on). In these changed times, the right to welfare benefits has come to the foreground as people's fear of being forced into inappropriate jobs or having their benefits cut off has taken precedence.

At the outset I would like to make it clear that I am NOT arguing that everyone be forced to work in any job under a threat of withdrawal of benefits if they do not. However, I do believe that:

- The choice **not** to work is only a choice if the person **really** has the opportunity to gain employment and pursue their career should they so wish. There is a big difference between someone choosing to fast when they can access food and enforced starvation through lack of food.
- In order to ensure that everyone has a **real** choice to work they must have the right to all the support and adjustments they need, for as long as they need them, in order to make a success of employment – the same right to accessible workplaces that people with other impairments have fought for and that are enshrined in the United Nations Convention on the Rights of Persons with Disabilities (2006). At present this right is denied to the majority of people with a mental health condition. We have much to learn from, and much to gain from being a part of, the broader disability movement with its social model of disability and rights based campaigning.
- No-one with a mental health condition is intrinsically unemployable. Everyone has something to contribute to the communities in which they live and could work at least some of the time in the right job with the right kind of support and adjustments. The fluctuating and long term nature of some mental health conditions may mean that some people can only work intermittently and/or with a very high level of support. If they

are to be denied the right to contribute their talents because the support they need is not available this is a **political** decision, not a 'clinical' one.
♦   Many people with mental health conditions currently work in a range of voluntary capacities, including training, political activism and advocacy. Volunteering undoubtedly has a place, but not when it is an enforced alternative to paid employment. I consider it to be exploitation if people with a mental health conditions do not have the opportunity to be properly recognised via payment (at the going rate for the job – not paltry 'therapeutic earnings') for the valuable contribution they make.

Why employment?

Recognition of the importance of work is not new. As far back as 172AD the Greek physician and philosopher Galen described employment as *'nature's best* physician' and *'essential for human happiness'*. The value of work is one of the few areas on which people coming from very different theoretical perspectives can agree. Freud said that people need two things – love and work – and that it is work which *'binds the individual to reality'*. Thomas Szasz describes work as *'the closest thing to a panacea known to medical science'* (see Rowland & Perkins, 1988). More recently, perhaps the clearest message comes from Professor of Psychiatry Bob Drake:

> In following people for 30 years and then following patients who are in dozens and dozens of research studies that are sent around, it's totally clear to me at this point that there's nothing about medications or psychotherapies or rehabilitation programs or case management programs or any of the other things that we study that helps people to recover in the same way that supported employment does. (Drake, 2008)

But testimony to the value of work comes not only from within the health diaspora. Eighteenth century poet William Cowper, who himself experienced periods of mental illness throughout his life and was confined to an asylum for over a year, considered that *'the absence of occupation is not rest, a mind quite vacant is a mind distressed'* while 20th century American novelist William Faulkner remarked that work is *'just about the only thing that you can do for eight hours a day'*.

It has become fashionable to talk about the stress of work and working in an unsuitable environment can be harmful (Warr, 1987), although the negative effects of high demand situations can be mitigated by support in the work setting and the employee having control over their work (Karasek, 1979; North et al, 1996). However, repeated research demonstrates that the stress of unemployment can be far more deleterious to health and well-being (see Rowland and Perkins, 1988; Royal College of Psychiatrists, 2002; Waddell & Burton, 2006; the Cross Government National Mental Health and Employment Strategy, 2009 and Perkins et al, 2009 for a summary).

If you are unemployed you are more likely to develop a range of physical health problems and die prematurely. This is serious as we know that people with more serious mental health conditions have a life expectancy some 10 years less than those without (Disability Rights Commission, 2006). However, there is a particularly strong relationship between unemployment and mental health difficulties. Unemployment brings with it an increased risk of a person developing a mental health condition, increased risk of relapse and re-hospitalisation if you already have such a condition, and increased risk of suicide.

As well as providing us an income that enables us to do the other things we value in life, work gives us a meaning and purpose in life – a reason to get up in the morning – and a means of structuring our time. It provides us with a sense of personal achievement, status and identity in society and social contacts. We are most likely to meet our friends and partners in the course of our work or education. Instead of using the extra time that unemployment brings for social and leisure pursuits, unemployment is associated with a decrease in social contacts and a decrease in activity (Jahoda et al, 1933). The existence of work in a person's life is a necessary counterpoint to leisure: without work - the things we have to do - the concept of free time and leisure has no meaning (Rowland & Perkins, 1988).

Most of all, work links us to the communities in which we live. It allows us to do things for other people and have our contribution recognised in the form of payment, which in turn provides a sense of personal achievement and self-worth.

Whether we like it or not, our jobs in large part define status and identity in society. Any class of person – like people with mental health conditions – that is routinely excluded from the labour market is therefore devalued, marginalised and excluded from the 'warp and weft' of everyday life. For people who are already excluded because of their mental health condition, work takes on an even greater importance. Those of us with mental health conditions are particularly sensitive to the isolation, loss of identity, structure and purpose that unemployment brings. Unemployment can so easily lead to loss of all identities other than that of 'mental patient' and reinforces the notion that we have little (if anything) to contribute.

Recovery and work: The chance to contribute

Everyone who experiences a mental health condition faces the challenge of recovery: living with and growing beyond what has happened. We have to re-evaluate our lives, work out what is important to us, find and use our own personal resources and resourcefulness in order to rebuild a new sense of who we are and of meaning and purpose in our lives. The status, identity, meaning and purpose afforded by employment can be critical.

There is no way back to how we were before ... but many people who have faced the challenge of life with a mental health condition have shown us that there is a way forward. Recovery is possible.

> [Recovery is] ... a way of living a satisfying, hopeful and contributing life, even with the limitations caused by illness. Recovery involves the development of new meaning and purpose in life as one grows beyond the catastrophic effects of mental illness. (Anthony, 1993 cited in New Horizons, 2009).

> Recovery is a process of healing ... of adjusting one's attitudes, feelings perceptions, beliefs, roles and goals in life. It is a painful process, yet often one of self-discovery, self-renewal and transformation. Recovery is a deeply emotional process. Recovery involves creating a new personal vision for one's self. (Spaniol et al, 1997).

Everyone's journey of recovery is personal and unique yet the accounts of people who have embarked on this journey reveal three things that appear to be particularly important (Repper and Perkins, 2003; Perkins, 2006; Shepherd et al, 2008): hope, control and opportunity ,... and in all of these, work has a role to play.

Hope and hope-inspiring relationships

> The turning point in my life was... where I started to get hope. Dr. Charles believed that I could. And Rev Goodwin believed that I could. Certain people believed that I could... and held that belief even when I didn't believe in myself. (Vincent, 1999)

It is not possible to move beyond what has happened and rebuild a life for yourself unless you believe that a decent life is possible. In the face of what seem like insurmountable odds – not least the myths and prejudice that surround mental health conditions – too many people have given up on themselves and their possibilities: resigned themselves to an existence on the margins of society or been unable to find any reason for continuing to live. Hopelessness can be fatal.

> 'For those of us who have been diagnosed with mental illness and who have lived in sometimes desolate wastelands of mental health programmes, hope is not just a nice sounding euphemism. It is a matter of life and death. (Deegan, 1988)

Relationships are central to holding on to hope. There are times when all of us find it difficult to believe in ourselves and our possibilities and we need someone else to believe in us, hold on to hope for us. It is difficult to believe in yourself if everyone around you thinks you will never amount to very much. But if that hopelessness is reflected in mental health services then this is doubly damaging: if the experts don't think I will ever amount to very much, what hope is there?

The stereotypes prevalent in society do little to inspire hope. Basically, if you have a mental health condition, you have two options: you can either be unpredictable and dangerous, or incompetent and unable and unfit to participate fully in society. Sadly, these ideas so prevalent in a wider society are reflected in mental health services.

The introduction to the National Service Framework for Mental Health (Department of Health, 1999) stated that 'most people who suffer from mental illnesses are vulnerable and present no threat to anyone but themselves' but that 'the small minority of mentally ill people ... are a nuisance or a danger to both themselves and others.'

Professional literature and research of all hues is replete with accounts of risk, deficit and dysfunction.

> ... even the briefest perusal of the current literature on schizophrenia will immediately reveal to the uninitiated that this collection of problems is viewed by practitioners almost exclusively in terms of deficit dysfunction and disorder. A positive or charitable phrase or sentence rarely meets the eye ... (Chadwick, 1997)

On the one hand, such a perspective has a profoundly negative impact on the attitudes and practices of mental health workers.

Deficit-obsessed research can only produce theories and attitudes which are disrespectful of clients and are also likely to induce behaviour in clinicians such that service users are not properly listened to, not believed, not fairly assessed, are likely treated as inadequate and are also not expected to be able to become independent and competent individuals in managing life's tasks.' (Chadwick, 1997)

On the other hand, the impact of a focus on the deficits, dysfunctions and disorder of people with mental health conditions also serves to shape and reinforce prevailing constructions of 'madness' in our society ... including the belief that people with mental health conditions are unlikely to be able to work at all, let alone pursue successful careers. This contributes to the maintenance of negative attitudes towards people with a mental health condition among the public in general and employers in particular. It also erodes the hope and possibilities of those of us diagnosed with such conditions. Forever emphasising risks, dangers, deficits and dysfunctions saps people of the strength they need to overcome the challenges they face and erodes the hope that are is central to recovery.

Taking back control over your life, your problems and the help you receive

To me recovery means being in the driving seat of my life. I don't let my illness run me. Over the years I have worked hard to become an expert in my own self-care. Over the years I have learned different ways of helping myself. Sometimes I use medications, therapy, self-help, mutual support groups, friends, my relationship with God, work, exercise, spending time in nature – all of these measures help me remain whole and healthy even though I have mental health problems. (Deegan, 1993)

When you develop a mental health condition you are surrounded by experts. Too often everyone you meet – within and outside mental health services – seems to think they know better what you think, feel and need than you do yourself, believes they know what is best for you: 'You should ...', 'You ought not to ...', 'The best thing to do is ...'.

I can talk, but I may not be heard. I can make suggestions, but they may not be taken seriously. I can voice my thoughts, but they may be seen as delusions. I can recite my experiences, but they may be interpreted as fantasies. To be an ex-patient ... is to be discounted. (Leete, 1988)

Recovery involves taking back control: becoming an expert in your own self-care and deciding what helps you in your recovery journey and deciding what you want to do in life: your personal dreams and ambitions rather than those that other people think would be 'good for you'.

People may have many goals and ambitions in life, but for most people, three things are critical: jobs, homes and friends - something to do, somewhere to live, and someone to love. Starting or re-starting your working career can be important in and of itself, but it can also be important in:

+ providing the resources you need to set up the home you want,
+ meeting people and finding someone to love,
+ affording you financial autonomy by reducing your dependence others for your income, and
+ increasing the range of choices available to you.

Opportunity: the chance to become more than just a mental patient and do the things you value in life

> Though a simple aspiration for most people socially isolated by mental illness, the sense of belonging to a community with all this can imply for mutuality and participation remains stubbornly elusive in spite of community care. (Morris, 2001)

It is impossible to rebuild your life – develop a new sense of meaning, purpose and identity within and beyond what has happened to you – if everywhere you turn you are debarred from doing the things you want to do. Those of us with mental health conditions, like other disabled people, have a right to those opportunities that all citizens should take for granted: to be a valued part of our communities, to enjoy all those opportunities available in those communities, and most importantly, the chance to contribute to those communities.

Too often, those of us with mental health conditions end up on the receiving end of help from everyone else ... even our parents and partners are mysteriously transformed into 'carers' with all the loss of that reciprocity that this implies (Perkins, 2001). Always being on the receiving end of help and hand outs from others is dispiriting and devaluing place to be. We gain our sense of value and self-worth not by receiving help, but by giving it. Employment is an important, probably the most important, socially valued and validated way in which we can contribute to our communities. Work is the means via which we do things for other people and are rewarded for our endeavours via being paid.

It boosts self-esteem and provides a sense of purpose and accomplishment. Work enables people to enter, or re-enter, the mainstream after psychiatric hospitalisation. (Rogers, 1995).

A job defines you, provides money, social networks, relationships, confidence, satisfaction, personal fulfilment and a sense of achievement. This is what I am, and this is what I do, I am no longer a mental health condition.

Over a year later I am still working successfully. I now focus more on opportunities in life and less on my condition. I regularly socialise with my colleagues after work and actually feel content to be a tax-payer again... He [employment support specialist] has enabled me to make the journey towards recovery and realise my aim of contributing to society again through fulfilling employment. (Perkins et al, 2009)

Having a job helps people to feel part of mainstream family and community life.

It's so good. My husband and daughter go out at 8.30am and I was the one left behind. Now we all go out together. (Perkins et al, 2009).

Now I have something to talk about with the family at Sunday lunch time. (A secretary talking about her first job for 8 years).

It was great to be in the tube in the rush hour. All those people, I finally feel part of life again.' (A man who had spent six of the previous ten years in a psychiatric hospital).

And we should never underestimate the impact symbolic value of being paid for your efforts. I have seen many tears shed over the first pay cheque a person receives after years of unemployment. As one woman said to me:

It was an amazing feeling. The first time anyone had paid me for something I had done for 15 years. I had done voluntary work but I never felt I would be able to do anything worth paying for again.

What denies us the right to work?

Often people cite the symptoms, deficits and dysfunctions that are reputed to accompany the diagnosis of a mental health condition as evidence that those of us with such conditions are incapable of work. Yet everywhere I see people with mental health conditions – including those who have what have been termed 'severe and enduring mental illnesses' - involved in a wide array of voluntary work, mutual support, campaigning, political activism, and a whole range of peer training and 'user involvement' activities. However, they are often paid on a casual and paltry basis with none of the pensions, sick pay and other benefits that those providing services receive. It is a myth that people with mental health conditions have nothing to contribute – and a travesty of justice that so often they do not receive proper recognition in the form of payment for so doing and all the benefits that employment brings.

Numerous research endeavours have failed to demonstrate a clear relationship between diagnosis, longevity or severity of mental health conditions and employment outcomes if people have the right kind of support and adjustments. Just like people with physical, mobility and sensory impairments and a range of long term health conditions, the most important factors determining whether we can get a job are whether we believe that we are capable to work (a belief that is readily eroded by the scepticism of those around us) and whether we are provided with the support and adjustments that we need to make a success of our employment (see, for example, Anthony 1994; Bond et al 2004).

We know that empowerment and access to employment are central to the recovery of many people (Warner, 2010). Yet the reality is that popular myths and stereotypes about people with a mental health condition – both within and outside services - result in fear, low expectations. These, when combined with a failure to provide the support and adjustments that people need, combine to produce a conspiracy of hopelessness: a vicious cycle to that denies all but a fortunate few the right to paid employment.

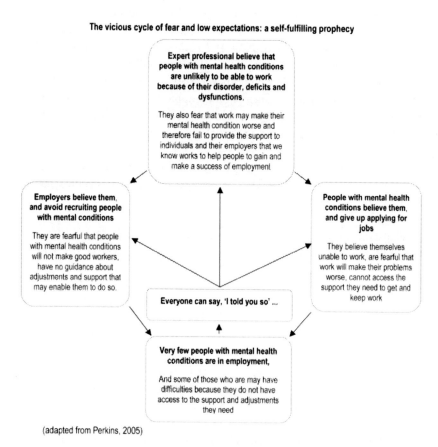

The vicious cycle of fear and low expectations: a self-fulfilling prophecy

(adapted from Perkins, 2005)

Fear and low expectations

Too many people have had their hopes and dreams dashed by the gloomy professional prognoses, and nowhere is this more evident than in the arena of work (Social Exclusion Unit, 2004). In one study, 40% of people with a mental health condition who were in employment had been told by a mental health professional that they could never work again (Rinaldi, 2000), and they were the ones who had been 'non-compliant' – got jobs in the face of professional judgments that they could not work. How many people believe the professionals and give up any thought of working?

> I'd love to go back to work ... earning your own money, being your own person ... but they won't let me back. The GP and the doctors at the hospital say 'no'. (Repper et al, 1998)

> When I said I wanted to work I was told this was an unrealistic goal. That I was too sick and the stress would be too much. I ... gave up any idea of work ... I lived with no hope of a future.

> My doctor told me I would never work again, eventually you start believing what they are saying.

> I have had two medical assessments – one lasted 2 minutes the other lasted 5 minutes. [Each time] the doctor opened my file, saw I was on lithium, closed the file and ended the assessment. He assumed I couldn't work because I am bipolar. (all cited in Perkins et al, 2009).

The low expectations of mental health professionals are communicated to both people with mental health professionals and employers resulting in a vicious cycle of low expectations. On 'expert' advice, people with mental health conditions come to believe themselves as incapable of working and therefore give up applying for jobs. Employers believe them incapable of working and avoid recruiting them. This ensures that very few people with mental health conditions are successful in employment ... and everyone's beliefs that people with mental health conditions are unable to work are reinforced. This vicious cycle of low expectations is reinforced by a vicious cycle of fear.

Many mental health workers, from the best of motives, may discourage those with whom they work from seeking employment because:

- They fear that it may worsen their mental health condition they fear it will worsen their mental health, financial position.
- They fear that people will be rendered worse off financially if they get a job because of the 'benefits trap'. Most mental health workers are not welfare rights experts and are ignorant of the complex array of welfare to work and in-work benefits. They are therefore not in a position to provide accurate information to their worried clients and frequently offer advice not to 'rock the boat' by seeking employment. It is true that the benefits system is far from perfect, but recent years have seen a number of improvements which mean that most people are better off in work (see Perkins et al, 2009) however, the complexities and inefficiencies in the system make it very difficult for anyone to navigate unaided so expert advice and guidance is of the essence.
- They fear that people will fail because of both their problems and the prejudice and discrimination that exist. There is a widely held belief that people with mental health conditions should be protected from failure, but in reality there is dignity in risk and recovery – rebuilding your life – inevitably involves taking risks. If mental health workers are to help people in their journey of recovery the challenge is not to protect people from, but support people in taking the risks that will enable them to explore their possibilities and rebuild their lives.

Only a Person who Risks is Free
by Author Unknown

To laugh is to risk appearing the fool.
To weep is to risk appearing sentimental.
To reach for another is to risk involvement.
To expose your ideas, your dreams,
before a crowd is to risk their loss.
To love is to risk not being loved in return.
To live is to risk dying.
To believe is to risk despair.
To try is to risk failure.
But risks must be taken, because the
greatest hazard in life is to risk nothing.
The people who risk nothing, do nothing,
have nothing, are nothing.
They may avoid suffering and sorrow,
but they cannot learn, feel, change,

grow, love, live.
Chained by their attitudes they are slaves;
they have forfeited their freedom.
Only a person who risks is free.
(in Gadsby, 2000)

These fears of professionals are communicated to people with mental health conditions, who may already be anxious about returning to work because of the negative experiences and lack of support they may have had in the past. Media images of 'social security scroungers' and threats of loss of benefits only exacerbate these fears and make it less likely that people will feel able to seek employment or be able to do so.

It is not therefore surprising that the suggestion that they might be able to work strikes fear into the hearts of many people with mental health conditions: better to remain in the secure poverty of life on welfare benefits – with all the negative implications that unemployment brings for health and well-being - than take the risk of seeking work.

But fear is not restricted to people with mental health conditions and the services designed to provide them with their treatment and support. Potential employers fear that people with mental health conditions will be inefficient and disruptive in the work place. In reality, many of the supports and adjustments that employers can make to enable people with a mental health condition to work successfully are similar to those which might enhance the performance of everyone in employment (see Perkins et al, 2009). Given the prevalence of mental distress, many will have had friends or relatives who have had 'a breakdown' or 'trouble with their nerves', or have experienced such difficulties themselves. However, the fear engendered by mysterious psychiatric labels and the catalogues of deficit, disorder and dysfunction that surround them lead many to fear that they will not have the expertise or resources to deal with any difficulties that do arise. Better not to take the risk.

Failure to provide appropriate support

The vicious cycle of fear and low expectations that denies people with mental health conditions the right to work is further exacerbated by a failure to provide support: the sort of support that repeated research shows can help the majority of people with mental health conditions to get and keep work – even those with more 'severe' and enduring' mental health difficulties.

There are now at least 16 'randomised controlled trials' across the world which show that if we provide people with the right kind of support 'Individual Placement and Support,' an average of 60% of people with a mental health condition can get and keep work (see Burns et al, 2007; Bond et al, 2008; Sainsbury Centre for Mental Health, 2009).

In the UK, two beliefs are widespread:

+ Treatment should precede any attempts at helping people with employment: we should first treat a person's symptoms and only then think about vocational rehabilitation.
+ People should start in a sheltered, supported setting where they can develop their skills and confidence before taking the plunge into the real world of work – open employment.

These may seem like 'common sense', but all of this research shows that it may not make as much sense as is commonly believed (Bond et al, 2008). The research evidence clearly shows that there are seven key principles of effective employment support (Bond et al., 2004):

+ Treatment and employment support must be offered in parallel. Employment Specialists must be integrated into clinical treatment teams and employment support must be an integral component of treatment and support plans.
+ People should not be selected on the basis of 'employability' or 'work readiness' – anyone who wants to explore the possibility of working should be assisted to do so.
+ Our focus must be on 'real work' – helping a person to gain and /or retain open employment rather than sheltered work. Work in sheltered settings does not increase people's chances of gaining open employment.
+ We should help people to get jobs that are in line with their interests and preferences rather than what professionals feel would be good for them.
+ People should be assisted to get a real job as quickly as possible with minimal pre-vocational training – any such training or work experience should occur in parallel with job search. Ongoing in-work training can then help people to pursue their careers.
+ Support for both the individual and their employer should be tailored to the person's needs and should be available without limit of time. A key feature of many mental health conditions is that they often fluctuate, therefore support needs to be flexible and available for as long as the person needs it.

> ♦ We must make sure that people have access to expert advice on welfare to work and in-work benefits to assist them through the transition to work and allay fears of financial insecurity during the process.

We must also recognise the importance of peer support – the hope, advice and images of possibility that people can gain from others who have made a similar journey and the importance of helping people to become experts in their own self-care. This can be achieved by using 'Wellness and Recovery Action Plans' for work or similar self-management approaches that can help people to work out how to keep themselves well at work and manage difficulties that may arise. Such approaches can also address adjustments that the employer might make and ways in which the employer, and other supporters, can assist the person in these endeavours (see Perkins et al, 2009).

Sadly very few people have access to the sort of support that we know can help them in their journey to work. Perhaps this is because many mental health workers are ignorant of the research evidence. Or maybe - because of the deep-seated prejudice and images of deficit and dysfunction that surround mental health conditions - other mental health workers simply do not believe the research evidence, or think that it does not apply to 'their' clients.

However, there may be more fundamental difficulties arising from the 'treatment, cure and care'; approach that guides the work of most health and social services.

Changing the terms of debate: Learning from the broader disability world

Health and social services typically view mental health conditions as 'illnesses'. As with other illnesses this means it is often assumed that should be 'tucked up in bed'- receive treatment and refrain from work and the responsibilities of everyday life. Until you are 'better' you should receive 'care' and be relieved of your responsibilities. This is fine for time-limited 'illnesses' – however the reality is that many mental health conditions – whether they be 'common' or 'severe,' fluctuate ... and some are ever present. For those of us with longer term or recurrent conditions the effect of this 'treatment, cure and care' approach is to relieve people indefinitely of the roles and responsibilities that give our lives meaning, purpose and value. The role of 'mental patient', or 'service user/survivor' eclipses all other identities.

If those of us with mental health conditions are to enjoy the rights and responsibilities of citizenship I believe we have much to learn from the social model of disability that guides thinking and action in the broader disability arena (see Perkins and Rinaldi, 2010). A social model of disability argues that people are not disabled by their impairments but by the way in which our communities fail to provide the supports and adjustments that the person needs to do the things they want to do, live the life they want to lead and enjoy those opportunities that all citizens should take for granted. A person with a broken spine is not disabled by being unable to use their legs, they are disabled by failure to provide supports (like a wheelchair), assumptions that everyone is able to stand and walk (like high work surfaces and steps) and the prejudice and stereotypes that have historically meant that people with mobility impairments are considered 'poor unfortunates' who are unable to participate fully in community life.

> Although treatment to minimise distressing and disabling symptoms is important this does not constitute an end in itself. Nor is it a necessary or sufficient condition for employment. For example, even if a person's symptoms can be permanently eliminated, that person remains disabled by the prejudice that surrounds someone with a history of mental health problems. Also, if a person has episodic or ever present 'symptoms' this does not mean that they cannot work or enjoy other citizenship opportunities, but they may require support and assistance to do so. (Perkins & Rinaldi, 2010)°

A social model of disability shifts the focus from 'changing the person so that they fit in' to 'changing the world so it can accommodate the person'. Such an approach has resulted in disability discrimination legislation, initially in the form of the Disability Discrimination Act (1995) and more recently the Equality Act (2010) as well as the United Nations Convention on the Rights of Persons with Disabilities (2006). These enshrine in law disabled people's rights to the support and adjustments they need to live full and independent lives. In theory, these rights explicitly extend to those of us with mental health conditions - in practice, the focus has often been on people with physical impairments. The right to 'treatment' and 'care' is not enough: it is the right to a life - full citizenship - that we need and to which we should be entitled ... including the real choice to work.

If, alongside other disabled people, those of us with mental health conditions are to enjoy such rights it is vital to insist that equal attention be placed on the sorts of support and adjustment that we need to make this vision a reality. Typically when we think about 'disability access' we think about the adjustments and supports that some people need to access the physical environment (ramps, hearing loops, wheelchairs, lowered work surfaces). Those of us with mental health conditions need adjustments and supports that can accommodate the fluctuation in our conditions and the impact that they can have on our ability to negotiate the social (as opposed to the physical) world.

In relation to employment this might include:

+ flexible provision of support in the workplace and temporary adjustments in work expectations to accommodate fluctuations in our condition (I myself need to be excused meetings at times),
+ easy access to more intensive treatment and support outside work when we need it, and
+ providing both employer and employee with financial security during periods when we are unable to work: a benefits system that allows people to move flexibly between work and welfare and funding to enable employers to bring in temporary cover when we are unable to work so that our jobs remain open to us.

But most of all we must raise our expectations.

Daring to dream

No-one with a mental health condition is intrinsically unable to contribute to our communities via employment. Everyone has talents to offer. Everyone can contribute IF they have the support and adjustments they need to do so. Some people may only be able to work episodically, others may only be able to work with a great deal of support – maybe needing someone with them all of the time ... and remember, there are people with mobility and sensory impairments who have 'personal assistants' with them at all time so that they can work and pursue their lives.

It is not mental health conditions that deny people citizenship and the right to contribute to our communities via work, but a vicious cycle of low expectations and failure to provide the support and adjustments needed. It may be that the state decides that there is a limit to the level of adjustments and support that our society can afford to provide – but this is a political or economic decision not a clinical one. It is also an issue of the use of scarce resources. For example, the 'Access to Work' budget is designed to fund the adjustments and support disabled people need at work. It is, quite simply, unjust that less than 1% of this budget goes to support people with a mental health condition in work (see Perkins et al, 2009).

If those of us with mental health conditions are to live the lives we want to lead and have access to those opportunities and choices that everyone should expect we must raise our expectations – keep daring to dream.

Believe in our possibilities and demand those rights - including the right to the support and adjustments we need to work and pursue our careers - that are enshrined in the United Nations Convention on the Rights of Persons with Disabilities.

> It's simple – we want disabled people to have a great start to life with equal access to education and play. We want disabled people to find work, have interesting careers and access to training.
>
> We want disabled people to have equality in their everyday lives: getting around on public transport, living in housing that meets their needs, and accessing goods and services.
>
> We want disabled people to enjoy their social lives: have families and friends, take part in sports and leisure activities, and serve the community. (Office for Disability Issues, 2009).

References

Anthony W. (1994) Characteristics of people with psychiatric disabilities that are predictive of entry into the rehabilitation process and successful employment. *Psychosocial Rehabilitation Journal,* 17: 3–13.

Anthony, W. (1993) Recovery from mental illness: The guiding vision of the mental health system in the 1990s. *Innovations and Research,* 2, 17-24.

Bird, L. (2001) Poverty, social exclusion and mental health: a survey of peoples' personal experiences. *A Life in the Day,* 5, 3, 4-8.

Bodman, R. et al. (2003) *Life's Labours Lost. A study of the experiences of people who have lost their occupation following mental health.* London: The Mental Health Foundation.

Bond, G.R. et al (2007) An update on randomised controlled trials of evidence-based supported employment. *Psychiatric Rehabilitation Journal,* 31, 208-289.

Bond, G.R. et al, (2004) Supported employment: Evidence for an evidence-based practice, *Psychiatric Rehabilitation Journal,* 27, 345-359.

Burns, T.et al, (2007) The effectiveness of supported employment for people with severe mental illness. A randomised controlled trial, *The Lancet*, 370, 1146-1152.

Chadwick, P. (1997) *Schizophrenia: The positive perspective. In search of dignity for schizophrenic people*, London: Routledge.

Clothier, C. (1994) *The Allitt Inquiry*. London: HMSO.

Cross Government (2009) *Working our way to better mental health. A framework for* action. London: Department of Work and Pensions.

Deegan, P. (1988) Recovery: The lived experience of rehabilitation. *Psychosocial Rehabilitation* Journal, 11, 11-19.

Deegan, P. (1993) Recovering our sense of value after having been labelled mentally Ill. *Journal of Psychosocial Nursing and Mental Health Services*, 31, 7-11.

Department of Health (1999) *National Service Framework for Mental Health*. London: Department of Health.

Department of Health (2009) *New Horizons: Towards a shared vision for mental health consultation*. London: Department of Health.

Disability Rights Commission (2006) *Equal Treatment: Closing the Gap*. London: Disability Rights Commission.

Drake, R.E. (2008) *The Future of Supported Employment. Sainsbury Centre Lecture, March 2008* www.scmh.org.uk/employment/services.aspx

Gadsby, J. (2000) *Addiction by Prescription*. Canada: Parker Books.

Galloway, J. (1991) *The Trick is to Keep Breathing*. London: Jonathan Cape.

Jahoda, M., Lazersfeld, P. & Zeisl, H. (1933) *Marienthal: The Sociography of an Unemployed Community*. London: Tavistock Publications.

Karasek, R. (1979) Job demands, job decision latitude and mental strain: implications for job redesign. *Administrative Science Quarterly*, 24, 285-308.

Leete, E. (1988) The treatment of schizophrenia: A patient's perspective. *Hospital and Community Psychiatry*, 38, 486-491.

Morris, D. (2001) Citizenship and community mental health. A joint national programme for social inclusion and community partnership. *The Mental Health Review*, 6, 21-24.

Office for Disability Issues (2009) *Roadmap 2025. Achieving disability equality by 2025*. London: TSO www.odi.gov.uk

Perkins, R. & Rinaldi, M. (2010) Changing the terms of the debate: mental health and employment. In P. Gregg & G. Cooke Ed *'People are the principle agents of change in their lives ...' Liberation Welfare*. London: Demos, Open Left Project.

Perkins, R., Rinaldi, M. & Hardisty, J. (2010) Harnessing the expertise of experience: Increasing access to employment within mental health services for people who have themselves experienced mental health problems. *Diversity in Health and Care*, 7, 13-21.

Perkins, R., Farmer, P. & Litchfield P. (2009) *Realising ambitions: Better employment support for people with a mental health condition.* (A Review to Government Cm 7742) London: TSO.

Perkins, R. (2006) First person: 'you need hope to cope'. In Roberts, G., Davenport, S., Holloway, F. & Tattan, T. (Ed) *Enabling Recovery: The principles and practice of rehabilitation psychiatry,* London Gaskell.

Perkins, R. (2005) Is what we offer to patients half acceptable? Chapter 23, in C. McDonald, K. Schulze, R,M, Murray & M. Tohen (Eds) *Bipolar Disorder: Upswing in Research and Treatment.* Oxford: Taylor & Francis.

Perkins, R. (2001) Rejecting the concept of 'carer'. *Open Mind,* 109, 6.

Perkins, R. (1999) My three psychiatric careers. In P. Barker, P. Campbell & B. Davison (Ed) *From the Ashes of Experience: Reflections on Madness, Survival and Growth.* London: Whurr Publications.

Repper, J.M. & Perkins, R.E. (2003) *Social Inclusion and Recovery: A Model for Mental Health Practice.* London: Balliere Tindall.

Repper, J. Perkins, R. and Owen, S. (1998) 'I wanted to be a nurse....but I didn't get that far': women with severe ongoing mental health problems speak about their lives. *Journal of Psychiatric and Mental Health Nursing,* 5, 505-513

Rinaldi, M. (2000) *Insufficient Concern.* London: Merton Mind.

Rinaldi, M., McNeil, K., Firn, M., Koletsi, M. Perkins, R. & Singh, S. (2004) What are the benefits of evidence based supported employment for patients with first episode psychosis? *Psychiatric Bulletin, 28, 281-284.*

Rinaldi, M. and Perkins, R. (2007) Comparing vocational outcomes for two vocational services: Individual Placement and Support and non-integrated pre-vocational services in the UK. *Journal of Vocational Rehabilitation,* 27, 1, 21-27.

Rogers, J. (1995) Work is key to recovery. *Psychosocial Rehabilitation Journal,* 18, 5-10.

Rowland, L.A. & Perkins, R.E. (1988) You can't eat, drink and make love eight hours a day: The value of work in psychiatry. *Health Trends,* 20, 75-79.

Royal College of Psychiatrists (2002) *Employment Opportunities and Psychiatric Disability,* Council report CR111. London: Royal College of Psychiatrists.

Sainsbury Centre for Mental Health (2009) *Doing what works. Individual placement and support into employment,* London: Sainsbury Centre for Mental Health www.schm.org.uk

Shepherd, G, Boardman, J. & Slade, M. (2008) *Making Recovery a Reality,* London: Sainsbury Centre for Mental Health, www.scmh.org.uk

Social Exclusion Unit (2004) *Mental Health and Social Exclusion Report.* London: UK Office of the Deputy Prime Minister

Spaniol, L. et al (1997) Recovery from serious mental illness: what it is and how to assist people in their recovery. *Continuum,* 4(4), 3-15.

United Nations (2006) *Convention on the Rights of Persons with Disabilities.* www.

un.org/disabilities

Vincent, S.S. (1999) Using findings from qualitative research to teach mental health professionals about the experience of recovery from psychiatric disability In *Proceedings of the Harvard University Graduate School of Education Fourth Annual Student Research Conference*. Cambridge, MA, USA, 72-81.

Waddell, G. & Burton, A.K. (2006) *Is work good for your health and well-being?* London: TSO.

Warner, R. (2010) Recovery from schizophrenia and the recovery model. *Current Opinion in Psychiatry* 2009, 22:374–380.

Warr, P. (1987) *Work, Unemployment and Mental Health*. Oxford: Oxford University Press.

13
Recovery for practitioners: Stories to live by

Glenn Roberts

Glenn starts by reminding us of the power of stories and their rightful place in modern more evidence based psychiatry. He suggests that anthologies of service user stories invite us all to find a resonance with our own experiences 'in the company of others.' Indeed along with other colleagues from Devon, he has helped produce 'Beyond the Storms,' which is as beautifully illustrated as 'A Gift of Stories,' which he so admires. Having a story to tell is both a gift to ourselves and a way that 'we make our experience available to others.' He offers the readers two main stories in this chapter. The first is the story of the origins of medicine and the second his own story. He points out that the concept of the wounded healer finds its origins in the story of Chiron from Greek mythology. He comments, '... his wound was such that it would not heal and as an immortal he could not die and thus he became both the master of medicine and the original wounded healer...' Glenn's own story as a psychiatrist has had its own share of ups and downs. He shares with the reader his childhood origins in East London. Later in his professional life he became so low he tells us that at one point he 'sat up for three days and nights weighing up whether to hang myself from the noose I'd set up from a hanging basket from a skylight. It would undoubtedly have worked.' Yet surviving and coming through this dark period gave him the confidence 'to sit in the dark and on the edge with many others since.' Gifts of stories indeed.

Introduction: Where I'm coming from

I am very grateful to Gordon and Jerome for inviting me to offer a personal contribution to this gathering of hope and experience. I admire its ambition of offering vivid and inspiring descriptions of people struggling to find themselves in the context of their lives and seeking to create a place of connection beyond 'them and us'.

It's not the first time I've had an opportunity to offer a story of personal experience and recovery (Roberts, 2009) but a year on and starting from a different place, I find the story I have to tell has a different title, emphasis and ending. The past is of course immutable, but how we see it, what we make of it and how we live with it are constantly changing. New experiences offer new viewpoints and shifts of perspective and interpretation. Successive chapters in an unfolding story offer a re-evaluation of what has gone before. In contrast Arthur Klienman (1988) observed that, 'Chronicity arises in part from telling dead or static stories'. I take this to be a warning to all of us to remain curious and exploratory and to take care not to get 'caught in a story', particularly those of our own making.

As I approach the end of my clinical career I've been thinking a lot about how intimately interconnected my personal and working lives have been. Many people who become mental health practitioners are, like me, at least partly motivated by their personal and family experience which may have been painful and difficult but may also be a strength and a qualification. But this does not occur automatically and there is a need to find satisfactory ways of transforming personal experience into practical expertise available to our roles and responsibilities. There is a particular need to find a healing story (Roberts et al, 1999a), a way of thinking and speaking about our lives, which holds together our truths, our fractured selves, and enables us to become useful, hopeful and helpful to others.

It feels a tricky challenge to know just what to say, for life stories are not just stories about our lives but as alive-stories they define, inform and guide us. And I can hear the storyteller's warning to, 'take care about the stories you tell for you shall surely be lived by them.' How we say it is how we see it. So, in this chapter I offer an attempt to describe what I've found and learned in my search for stories-to-live-by that reconcile my personal experience and professional role in the hope that it may be useful to others but I also want to take care to preserve sufficient freedom of movement so I can keep my story alive and open to future changes too.

Valuing Stories

As I approach retirement I feel there still much to learn and I still regard my professional practice as, 'work in progress'. Perhaps this is inevitable when each day brings new encounters with unique circumstances and people deeply troubled by mysterious experiences, about which there are many theories but few, perhaps no, certainties. The broader picture is that after a century of research, severe mental health problems remain, fundamentally, of unknown origins – which doesn't mean we cannot be touched and moved and work for understanding, but that we do so primarily through stories.

Scientific medicine and psychiatry has, until recently, been little interested in stories and seen them as impediments to understanding, valuing objectivity and measurement over subjectivity and empathic connection. But that has and is changing rapidly and this depersonalised, some say dehumanised perspective, is giving way to re-evaluation of the need for meaning alongside measurement and passion alongside probability (Strauss, 1994; Greenhalgh and Hurwitz,1998; Roberts, 1999b, 2000).

Our conceptual and diagnostic frameworks give us shapes to look for and words with which to name the patterns that we see but meaning and understanding comes through stories, which offer a way of engaging with people, in context, over time. Conversely, we are impoverished if we lack a story of our personal and collective origins, where we have come from, our roots and relationships with what has gone before, and therefore who we are and where we belong.

Once we have eyes to see them we realize that we are surrounded by stories. We meet them in every newspaper and magazine, every TV programme and advertisement, each conversation about ourselves and one another. We construct them in our case conferences, reports and letters and exchange them in each handover and supervision and even in our gossip (Hunter, 1991). The storyographer Daniel Taylor (1996) goes so far as to say that, 'We live in stories the way fish live in water, breathing them in and out, buoyed up by them, taking from them our sustenance, but rarely conscious of this element in which we all exist. We are born into stories; they nurture and guide us through life.'

But the power of stories presents risks as well as opportunities and the master storyteller Chimamanda Adichie (2009) warns that there are many dangers when a single story comes to eclipse and dominate all others. Her discussion of 'the single story' is the story of stigma and stereotypes and how easily we define one another by particular characteristics which then restrict our vision and sense of possibility. She observes how the single story 'robs people of their dignity' and of the opportunity for people to find a way of belonging together in all their diversity. She concludes that, 'Stories matter. Many stories matter. Stories have been used to dispossess and malign but stories can also be used to empower and humanise. Stories can be used to break the dignity of a people but stories can also be used to repair that broken dignity'. And so the value of the present work is not only in the contributions of its authors but also the space in between them, that invites the reader to find a place for their story to be recognised and valued too.

The roots of the recovery movement in psychiatry (Davidson et al, 2010) can be traced back to humanistic philosophers, civil rights activists and compassionate clinicians over the last couple of hundred years, but it is the personal testimony of individuals that has fired and fuelled the contemporary recovery movement. Anthologies of personal recovery stories, such as Julie Leibrich's (1999) wonderful, *A Gift of Stories*, invites the reader to find resonance for their own experience in the company of others. This is built around the proposition that coming into one's own story, having a telling-tale, is both a gift to ourselves and a means by which we make our experience available to others and I've found this to be true.

By many people's standards I've lived a very stable and comfortable life with many rewards and much appreciation. I've also lived with a knowledge of how outward appearances and inner experiences can sometimes be markedly different and how alienating it can sometimes be to live with an awareness of gap and disconnection. Just as we are becoming interested to bridge the gap between 'them and us', 'staff' and 'patients', so there is a parallel consideration as to how we bridge the gaps between the strengths and vulnerabilities within ourselves and access sustaining stories that are hospitable to the breadth and complexity of our experience of life and work. These would be stories that enable us to be honest with ourselves and acceptable to others, without shame. Stories that support us in living and growing and becoming what we are able to be, so that we can author and if need be, re-author our lives (White and Epston, 1990). This applies as much to mental health practitioners as to people in recovery and of course many who are both at the same time.

So I'd like to offer two stories which are, for me, deeply inter-connected. One is drawn from my delving into the depths of the originating myths of my profession. The other is drawn from reflections on some of the more difficult experiences I've been through. Taken together they describe my attempts to seek out a sustaining story of how to reconcile my work with my life. Neither is of course anything like, 'the whole story' but I have learned to value them both and nowadays I feel satisfied with how well they get on with one another.

Restor(y)ing professionals:
The 'medical model' reconsidered ...

Being a doctor is so much more than a job. It is a contract of trust, a privilege, an education and an identity. Being a doctor in psychiatry is a complex and sometimes uncomfortable identity, with much said and felt about power, control, authority, responsibility and choice. In recent years I've found these discomforts amplified when drawn into debating the 'medical model' but diminished when working with others on the common purpose of supporting people in their recovery (CSIP et al, 2006). One can be a combative, accusatory even stigmatizing discourse, the other an orientation that centers on recognition that we are all 'people first' and values our shared humanity as the anchor point for all else.

Doctors, in particular psychiatrists, are often considered by others to be host and hostage to something called the 'medical model'. It is usually characterised as an excessive and unbalanced focus on conceptualising mental illness as due to people having 'broken brains' and needing biological (drug) remedies to correct 'the chemical imbalance'. Such a model of medicine is rightly seen as catastrophically reductive of both understanding and therapeutics for complex bio-psycho-social-cultural-existential (human) problems. It also is portrayed as a stigmatizing addition to people's burdens and an impediment to recovery. I also think it is wrong. A shallow caricature which undermines any appreciation of medical practice as fundamentally based on trusting relationships and doctors as people fundamentally concerned to relieve suffering and promote the wellbeing of their fellow human beings. And although I'm familiar with portrayals of such 'medical model' practitioners in drama and films, I cannot honestly say I've met them amongst my peers or colleagues.

I can understand how this has arisen from a skewed emphasis on psychiatry's eagerness to be scientific and be securely based on reliable 'evidence' and the dominance of pharmaceutical funding for research. But I also feel its ascendancy in critical discourse represents a disconnection with the longer and deeper story of medicine and the heartbeat of its origins. There is concern within psychiatry that, in this most personal area of medical practice, we have progressively depersonalized our writing, learning and teaching – at a considerable cost to all involved – including the medics, but that is changing (Bracken and Thomas, 2005).

As a trainee I had the good fortune to spend time with Dr Glin Bennet whose interest in the Jungian concept of the 'wounded healer' (Bennet, 1987) introduced me to a way of thinking about our personal struggles as practitioners that made them appear as potential qualifications rather than disqualifications. It also led to me thinking about how people live with their professional identity for good or ill and about the health needs of health practitioners (Rippere and Williams, 1985; Roberts, 1997). Digging a little deeper reveals that the origins of this concept are far more ancient and at the birth of this 'second oldest profession' we find stories of its founding fathers as ethicists, spiritual guides and dreamers all inspired by a mysterious wounded immortal, a Centaur, half man, half horse called Chiron. The traces and contribution of each remain with us today and in my view could helpfully be reclaimed as a contribution to the narrative foundation of our identity as practitioners.

The average pub quiz aficionado would reliably offer 'Hippocratic oath' as the answer to, 'What promise do doctors make on qualifying', although they don't nowadays and very few have even seen it. Those that do take a look at this 2500 year old charter for ethical practice may find it mighty strange. It begins

> I swear by Apollo the healer, Asclepius, Hygeia and Panacea, and I take to witness all the Gods, all the Goddesses, to keep according to my ability and my judgment, the following Oath and agreement.

It goes on to lay a solemn duty upon doctors to 'do no harm' such that, 'In every house where I come I will enter only for the good of my patients' and to preserve confidentiality as well as the integrity of medical practice.'

But where did Hippocrates, the 'Father of Western Medicine', learn it from? He tells us himself in this opening sentence of his mysterious oath. According to Greek myth, Hygeia ('Health') and Panacea ('Healing'), were daughters of Asclepius described by Homer as the 'exemplary physician' whose life and work led to the building of the some of the earliest 'hospitals' - dream temples and houses of healing staffed by physician priests. This included a famous temple at Kos, where Hippocrates learned and taught medicine. Snakes were revered as both agents of death and healing and Asclepius' snake entwined staff has been taken as the central icon of medicine and healing ever since.

Stepping back even further we learn from various stories that Asclepius was the son of the God Apollo and a mortal woman but began his life in tragedy, his mother having been killed by Apollo for unfaithfulness and he being cut from her belly on the funeral pyre. At birth he was given to the Centaur Chiron who had himself been raised by Apollo, and tracing the story of his origins takes us towards still older stories that underpin the whole of medicine. It is said that Chiron was born of a violent union of Chronos (Saturn) raping the sea nymph Philyra disguised in the form of a horse. His mother was so disgusted at the appearance of Chiron that she abandoned him at birth but he was rescued and raised by Apollo, God of poetry and music who schooled him in arts, sciences and mysteries. Chiron thus became different to his hedonistic and rowdy kin and became wisest amongst the Centaurs.

But one day he was accidentally wounded by Hercules with a deadly arrow dipped in Hydra blood. This was particularly tragic as Chiron had earlier prepared Hercules to successfully complete his 12 labours — heroic acts which live on as metaphors for the challenges facing each human being on the spiritual path. Some stories say that he invented medicine in an attempt to heal himself but his wound was such that it would not heal and as an immortal he could not die and thus he became both the master of medicine and the original wounded healer his vast knowledge of life being attributed to his vulnerability and his struggle with his own suffering.

Contemporary medicine therefore has deep in its ancestral roots, stories of forefathers who were illegitimate, despised and rejected, abandoned and raised by strangers. Creatures and people whose wounds were their wisdom and whose inheritance of empathy, spirituality, ethics and integrity continue to offer foundations for contemporary practice and practitioners. Improbable though it sounds there are resonances, words and images that continue to link us to this forgotten history wherever you look. There are many contemporary traces of Chiron's name to this day, including even in the basic qualifications of doctors, MB ChB., the Ch being derived from Chirology i.e. surgery. The Staff of Asclepius is the symbol of the British Medical Association and many other medical and paramedical bodies and the resurgence of interest in spirituality (Cook et al, 2009) harkens back to Asclepian dream temples and physician priests. And crucially, Hippocrates and his famous oath forever put medicine on an ethical foundation, the content of which is a very close parallel to today's definition by the General Medical Council of the fundamental 'duties of a doctor' (GMC, 2010).

So here is not so much a model of medicine as an interconnected series of foundational stories that connect contemporary practitioners with the image of the wounded healer, accepting our imperfection and vulnerability as an education. You can be strong and weak, wounded and wise – one does not disqualify the other so much as inform and enrich – humanise. Many who come into mental health work are at some level informed and motivated by their personal experience, (Roberts et al, 2011). For those that do there is an inevitable task of attending to your own healing, transforming your experience into expertise which can become as valuable as the knowledge you hold and the qualifications you have acquired. And hence one of the Key Challenges for future recovery oriented services is to 'support staff in their recovery journeys' (Shepherd et al, 2010).

Narrative transformations: Accommodating your experience

The narrative transition from victim to victor (Coleman et al, 2000), from patient to heroes and heroines (see Carson, Chapter 7) is an alchemical transformation that turns the leaden weight of our difficulties into something of great value that upholds us, attracts others and inspires hope. We are touched by personal stories of survival and overcoming which illustrate what it's like to have such experiences and light the path to recovery for others.

The transformation that is involved in reconstructing the story we live in may not only record changes in our lives but may constitute and consolidate those changes. The opportunity and freedom to live in a different story, to reconfigure the myth-we-live-by (Samuel and Thompson, 1990) can put the past into a different context. What looked like loss and waste can sometimes be re-evaluated as a wound that potentially holds wisdom and the beginning of something else. The transformational outcome of the lonely wanderings of the 'ugly duckling' was not in becoming a 'beautiful duckling' but in realisation that he was a swan and finding recognition and belonging amongst his own (Estes, 1992). Most people feel a need to belong and it is often through telling our telling-tales that we find our kin.

Speaking personally

Alongside thinking about the stories underpinning my work I've also been thinking about how to find value in some of the more difficult experiences of my life. It has taken me a long time to get to a place where I feel I have a clear view of what has gone before. I'm reminded of T S Eliot's humble and hopeful observation about later life that, 'We shall not cease from exploration. And the end of all our exploring will be to arrive where we started and know the place for the first time.' (Little Gidding).

I've known much success and have a great deal to be thankful for. But if I look back over my life I've often felt lost and disconnected. If we'd met in my early life I don't think I could have offered a coherent story at all. As youngster I was fairly sure I would die early – it turns out incorrectly. In middle life I would have given an inwardly preoccupied account overfull of tangles and sadness. Nowadays I feel I've largely come home to myself and reconnection with my family and I'm grateful with how life has worked out. This next section is a story of what I've recovered from and to and with.

For as far back as I can remember I've had periods of disabling depression, accompanied by a haunting sense of loneliness, detachment and isolation from people and the world around me. However it took me a long while to recognise it as such. Throughout my childhood and teenage years although frequently sad and fearful my experience was more of becoming unable to concentrate or do things for lengthy spells. I thought of it as a sort of hibernation. I just had to sit it out and needed to wait until I woke up again and could get on once more. I grew up with a story that my future career was predicted by a Gypsy who had rewarded my mother with a blessing rather than a cuss for buying a bunch of 'lucky white heather', and a prediction that her toddler would be a doctor - and the Gypsy was right, but it was a near thing.

The atmosphere in my family home was one of frequent dispute and arguments about trivial issues, there could be angry eruptions over who'd left the top off the tomato sauce. I only later realised how unhappy my parents were with one another. Perhaps understandably I was a naughty child, with little confidence who clung fearfully to anything that seemed to offer some security. From an early age I felt odd and different and later identified with being 'an outsider'. At about 8 I impressed an assessing psychologist sufficiently to be allocated a place in a residential school for disturbed boys. I'd largely forgotten this until much later when I had flashbacks visiting people in prison – the stairs in both were metal and clanged underfoot. I do remember being terrified and pleading to go home - my parents fought and nearly split up over it, but I escaped deportation to the 'naughty boys home'. I had a feeling of being on probation for the rest of my childhood. I still get a panicky sense of being in jeopardy and at risk of being abandoned resurfacing when I've been depressed.

I was slow to read and clumsy, nowadays I'd have a diagnosis and possibly help, back then I was just thought a bit stupid. Despite my difficulties one of my chief delights was to wrap up in the company of books, in particular the remaining 9 volumes of Arthur Mee's Children's Encyclopaedia. The mysterious volume 8 having been destroyed when my Father's childhood home was bombed in the war. These were full of wonders: how to make pets of all kinds of unsuitable creatures, glorious colour plates of birds and beetles and butterflies, and 'The great stories of the world that will be told forever' which I read over and over again. I spent much of my childhood wandering in Epping Forest. I was a sort of a feral nature-boy, in a middle class sort of way, with an Arthur Mee inspired disposition to catch anything that moved, in quantity.

I couldn't really relate to other children and was bullied. Looking back I can see that a principled but mouthy lad growing up in East London with no discernable athletic talent was liable to get into numerous fights and invariably lose. I may have attracted the playground predators but then I was waving a red flag at the time. My early school years came to be dominated by a sense of threat which I did my best to escape. As a young child I did this by bunking off and hiding in the garden amongst my father's dahlias and later into the cloistered world of laboratory assistants who, because of their 'duties', were never required to attend for assembly or register or much else come to that.

Despite the Gypsy's promise I was initially turned down by all the medical schools I applied to, probably due to having failing all my mock 'A' level exams and despite several attempts I'd still not gained English O level. I can look back now on my earlier failures with a wry smile, supported by multiple qualifications, national awards and nearly 60 published papers, but at the time it was a bit of a disaster as I had no other ideas about what to do with my life. Fortunately the ensuing panic was also highly motivational.

As a first year medical student I remember sitting up all night in a state of inexplicable excitement writing an essay on 'the self' based on a book about a young boy called Dibs who was crushed and contorted by the emotional disturbance within him to the point of being unable to communicate. The story of his opening and becoming thrilled me. I didn't realise at the time this was because of how much I saw myself in Dibs and longed for a similar release. I also thought psychiatry would be like that – working closely with people in great difficulties to find themselves – and I was disappointed, at least initially.

From my earliest student encounters with mental hospitals and their residents I felt in some measure at home. I was oddly comfortable with people who were distressed and disordered and found the surrealistic kaleidoscope of psychosis simply fascinating. The jokey rejoinder that, 'It takes one to know one', is not really as dismissive as it may at first appear – it may describe the difference between sympathy and empathy, listening and hearing, seeing and understanding, being professional and peer – and of course it is quite possible to do and be both but it's taken me a long time to reconcile this in my own life.

As a young psychiatrist I was very committed to the work but was stressed by the rush and pressure of working in acute settings and often felt overwhelmed. I was disappointed with the preoccupation with suppression rather than expression (most of our medical treatments are 'anti-something'), uncomfortable with the peculiar knowingness we are trained to profess about mysteries and rather oppressed by the claustrophobia of many of our clinical environments.

As a more senior psychiatrist I have been additionally frustrated with the ever present invitation to obsess over rearranging the organisational structures we work in rather than the work of developing creative outcomes and supporting hope for the people who come to us in need. Early on I developed a commitment to working in rehabilitation with people who have complex and often long term conditions. Over the years I've taken an interest in creative therapies, narrative perspectives, the pursuit of meaning and purpose and the role of applied drama in mental health education (Roberts et al, 2007). This has been balancing of the sometimes sombre responsibilities as I also have to treat people detained under the Mental Health Act. I've also had the good fortune to work in teams with many innovative and creative people particularly those from nursing and occupational therapy backgrounds with a deep and quiet commitment to the work. I've written elsewhere that working in psychiatry has been the making of me (Roberts, 2008) and for all its associated difficulty I hold that to be true. Working with supportive colleagues and people whose life problems in some measure overlap with my own has taken me on a maturational journey and looking back I can see that some routine clinical skills have enabled me to look after myself too.

Although I later became an examiner for the Royal College of Psychiatrists, I think I initially failed the Membership exams as I couldn't quite believe the received wisdom of my profession. Having eventually been persuaded to value science with its rigor and regularities, my preoccupation since has been in trying to reconcile that with the search for meaning and understanding. I have come to a personal belief, based on long experience, that every symptom tells a story and just because I cannot understand something doesn't mean it is nonsense.

Walking in the dark

Much of the underside of my adult life has been about struggling with depression. It is now much more acceptable to talk about it, although at times I've felt embarrassed and humiliated by my own experience. It is easily underrated by those who haven't been there. William Styron (1991) commented that, 'depression is a word that has slithered through the language like a slug, leaving little trace of its intrinsic malevolence.' He'd been there.

The experience of depression has many similarities from one person to another, but is also unique and coloured by who we are and how we live. So what's it been like for me? It is not just about a low mood, but the weighing down and running down of so much else as well, energy, hope, attention, concentration, capacity for life and relationships, and simply feeling wretched, ill and achy – not unlike flu but without the fever.

When well, I really enjoy driving along singing loudly to even louder 'dad-rock', but as I descend the first thing to go for me is any enjoyment of music which grates and jangles and I prefer both solitude and silence, although it is a silence increasingly populated by my own nagging thoughts of failure and uselessness. My usually overfull mind empties out and I feel I know nothing. I feel a boring fraud and a rising sense of threat and danger takes hold. Sleep and much else becomes difficult as the night fills with aching restlessness. The air thickens and everything becomes effortful, heavy and slow.

Moderate dips simply grind me down – I have to shut down for a bit, reprioritise and necessarily look after myself to regain my capacity to care for others. In recent years it's usually because I've overcommitted myself and a fuse has blown, sometimes it the only thing that makes me slow down or stop so maybe that is purposeful, if costly. Much as I try not to, I become very sensitive to actual or felt rejection – which is tricky as a mental health practitioner, but I've learned to question my own feeling-driven perceptions and try not to jump to conclusions. Longer periods feel increasingly precarious and with a haunting sense of danger and risk. I wake early with a sense of dread. I keep going but ordinary life can feel like skating on thin ice with an attendant fear of what would happen if I slowed down and fell into the inky depths beneath. I lose perspective and become afraid of people and withdraw from communication. It's easy to mistake feelings for facts. It seems to me that the world has changed, rather than I have and it can sometimes feel like living with a double reality and I'm not sure which is true.

Less frequently I've gone beyond that and it has felt that both I and the world around me are disintegrating. It is as though I can then see things as they really are; I do not feel I've become disordered so much as insightful. In depressive truth there is no hope or joy or love or purpose, it all appears to be an illusion that we create to cover up the emptiness and futility – the sheer pointlessness of life. Everything can seem out of control ... the growth of plants in the garden overwhelming, the cracks and imperfections in the house crumbling. I don't want to eat or sleep, everything slows and I don't say much. It is not a good place to be.

At my lowest I sat up for 3 days and nights weighing up whether to hang myself from a noose I'd set up for a hanging basket from a skylight. It would have undoubtedly worked. Thankfully it's not a place I've visited for some years now - although there is some tension even in remembering, like watching a horror movie that you are part of. In standing right on the edge and deciding 'no' I learned forever that you could get that close and still step back – which has given me confidence to sit in the dark and on the edge with many others since.

When depressed I long to be loved and valued and accepted, I long for closeness and connection with a deep ache – but at the same time I cannot easily accept kindness at face value. I feel I am shabby and unacceptable and feel that anyone with a real understanding of what I'm like would surely reject me. And so if you are kind and caring towards me it just shows how little you really know me – and so you are either not really relating to me at all or else not telling the truth – either way your kindness increases my sense of isolation and there is not a third way. I once found this well described in a book of poetry called 'Knots' by R D Laing.

A low turning point

I'd married young in search of security. Having never felt part of a family I had a naive longing to find or make one of my own. Ten years later and 'fully trained' we packed up our bags and 4 young children to move from inner city Bristol to a farmhouse in Devon with land and pets and assorted wildlife – and it was a delight. When we arrived I stood in the stream that bordered our land with my daughter and laughed and laughed at the joy of coming home. I'd come to North Devon on the 'small is beautiful' ticket and exchanged the paranoid politics of a large organisation for the 'periphery of excellence'. And it was good for many years, although later, as the organisation I worked in grew and grew, I was uncomfortable with the imposed requirement to relate to bigger and more remote structures.

In my early 40's my marriage failed. As our 4 children became more independent the somewhat unfathomable difficulties between us tangled beyond unravelling. Precarious communication broke down entirely. We tried very hard but even my own children could see the incompatibility of their parents and wondered why we were together. As our relationship broke down so did I, and entered what was possibly the most painful and disturbing period of my adult life. It took about 2 years before I properly emerged from that depression. With the loss of my marriage I lost much else besides, my home and imagined future, the daily love and challenge of my children, their cats and creatures, our lovely dog Tilley - and a good deal of my pride.

Living alone and unable to work or do anything much else, I spent that winter burning my way through a friend's wood pile, preoccupied with how everything I valued was also burning. I sat so still that for the first time in 25 years my self-winding watch stopped. After a few months with the kindly support of colleagues I made a cautious return to work – for the first time routinely wearing suits, 'body armour' as I joked, but I felt very vulnerable and loosely held together.

If I had to select one life experience that was the making of me – this was it – a traumatic induction into being real and joining the human race. It was a terrible and transformational time which now appears to have been the low turning point (Rakfelt and Strauss, 1989) around which my life pivoted and from which the future unfolded. If given a second mark to plot my recovery it would be unexpectedly finding Annie who was to become my wife. Twelve years later I still find myself married to my best friend and companion, the only person I've been comfortable to spend unending time with. We had both survived the breakdown of long marriages and, without looking, found one another. I've had a lot of good fortune but this was one of the best, a small miracle which has proven to be a secure foundation for love and life and living ever since.

Working for recovery

Recovery is work, often hard work. I'd agree with Jerome that the size of the task lies in proportion to the magnitude of the problem to be overcome and the availability of supports. But it is also quirky and just as we are familiar with bad things happening unexpectedly, so can good things too.

We also contribute to our own difficulties – at least I've found it so. One of the many things that make it difficult to recover is how attached we can become to our problems and how reluctant to give them up. I've found that there are seductive satisfactions in sadness and strangely consoling dark-pleasures in nurturing a sense of grief. It is really hard to let go of a sense of anger or resentment when you feel entitled to it, but holding onto it perpetuates these difficulties and when grief turns to grievance so does a little madness creep in. Not clinically recognisable psychosis but the madness of everyday life whereby you become convinced of truths and realities because you feel them so strongly. Giving it up, re-entering ordinary living is to encounter loss and re-encounter confusion and the realisation of having been mistaken. In my experience this is largely a relief, a sweet embarrassment to discover that although I felt shut out, it was really that I was pressing on a door that opens inwards. This transition, coming home to oneself and back into relationship with others, can be a humbling experience for which you need to draw on other sources of security to make the experience bearable – and clearly all the more difficult to face if you've little else to call on.

Personally I've only had to return from moderate depressive distortions and misinterpretations but the jolt has been sufficient to make me gasp at the magnitude of the re-evaluation that is involved in anyone recovering from long commitment to sincere errors of belief and understanding. The clinician may call this 'getting better' whereas the peer may see it more as a major task of reconstructing life and living. No wonder some find this 'awakening' a shock and struggle to cope with the pain and responsibility of recovery.

I've generally been more disposed to face my demons than run from them, which has also been the making of many adventures: fearing abandonment led to my hitchhiking around Europe alone - sleeping rough, fretful self-consciousness led to taking on frequent teaching and public speaking, my sense of existential confusion led to a doctoral thesis on meaning and purpose, and feeling alienated from my peers led to developing workshops and retreats on stress and burnout and setting up mentoring schemes. I've mostly found it helpful to be straightforward about my difficulties and experiences with the people I work with. The world has often proved to be a much kinder and more accepting place than I feel and fear when unwell.

I've learned slowly that if I don't look after my health and sanity I'm of little use to others, for you cannot give what you do not have. I've also learned to value my vulnerability. I was sad when my father died a few years ago but very glad to be so. For it was only in the context of my own difficulties in middle life that our relationship was remade sufficient for the sharing of tender feelings and a meaningful connection as men – and now I miss him and wish that he was still around – we could have gone fishing together.

Discovering 'recovery'

Reading and hearing accounts of personal recovery from the mid 1990s onwards resonated with what had drawn me into psychiatry in the first place. People spoke of finding hope in their journeys of personal discovery and of picking up responsibility for themselves and their lives - trying to work out what worked best for them on the basis of personal experience. I found this a hopeful and helpful approach that was equally applicable in my own life as for those I worked with. Annie and I moved to Exeter in 2003 and later that year I went with Laurie Davidson to learn about the Wellness Recovery Action Plan (WRAP) from Mary Ellen Copeland. This became pivotal to all our subsequent activity in Devon developing recovery ideas and practice. Learning about recovery pulled together so many of the threads from what had gone before and has been the most hopeful and helpful discovery of my 30 years in psychiatry. Here I found a story and a story of stories in which I could find a place for both my personal and professional experience and guiding values which saw each as supportive of the other.

The satisfaction of working in psychiatry is of helping people in great difficulties get over their problems and get on with their lives although you also need eyes to see it, for these kind of changes are sometimes very gradual with many a backwards step. But as people become committed to their own recovery and take authority over their lives such changes can gather pace and accumulate over time, sometimes years. This is why we chose 'Enabling Recovery' as the title for our guide to rehabilitation psychiatry (Roberts et al, 2006). Not that services can 'recover' anyone, but they can certainly help or hinder and we have much to learn from people's personal stories so as to do more of the former and less of the latter. I've become firmly convinced that 'enabling recovery' should be the aim and purpose of all mental health and social care services.

Over the last few years I've been closely involved with promoting a recovery approach in my NHS Trust and profession and working with the Sainsbury Centre's project on 'Making Recovery a Reality' (Shepherd et al, 2008). In particular I have contributed the view that a key challenge in 'Implementing Recovery' (Shepherd et al, 2010) includes, 'Supporting staff in their recovery journeys'. In Devon we conducted a survey of all staff working in the Trust and found that 43% of the 560 people who responded said they had personal experience of mental health problems and 63% of caring for someone close to them who had such difficulties (Roberts et al, in press). This supports a simple but radical observation – that 'staff' are people too and people attracted to working in psychiatry are likely to have had at least as much personal experience of mental health problems as the general population and quite probably a lot more. It also raises a hopeful possibility that people working in mental health services could be supported to transform this 'wealth of experience' into expertise available to those they seek to help (Daneault, 2008).

My discoveries in recovery have led me to hope for a future in which the training and development agenda for mental health workers is not only about developing skills in supporting others in their recovery but also about engaging in a recovery agenda for practitioners and the professions too. It points to a challenging and ambitious future for mental health practice where people are selected for their qualities as much as their qualifications. A future which engages with the person of the practitioner and their experience of life as well as supporting learning about research, evidence, critical appraisal and the limits of knowledge. As I approach the end of my career as a clinician I continue to have a hope for a future that supports a progressive process of cultural change that would enable all those working in mental health services not only to become technically competent but richly reconciled to their own humanity and increasingly able to be holders of hope, coaches, mentors and guides for people needing and seeking their help. I think this process of transformation has begun, and this book is a significant contribution to it. What becomes of this and how it works out in practice involves all of us and will include how you, the reader, respond to it ...

Postscript

Many things, people, situations and opportunities have helped me over the years and this is what I've learned to rely on – what works for me in supporting my life and health:

Work – being productive, making things and using my skills
Homemaking – nesting, holding together creativity and safety
Contemplation – study, thinking, writing, reading, talking, teaching
Medication – antidepressants and sleepers

Authenticity – valuing being real more than being comfortable
Apologising – accepting that I can get it wrong – saying sorry
Tenderness – being open to moments and places of real connection
Honesty – with myself and others – saying and facing things
Anchoring – rehearsing a conscious awareness of the people in my life whom I love and trust
Reaching out – connect and communicating with others - particularly when I don't feel like it
Practical usefulness – doing anything that needs doing
Giving – I feel better for giving to or seeking to be mindful of others
Prioritising – ordering, scheduling, listing, cancelling, delegating
Kindly realism – expecting less of myself when low so I can still succeed
Humour – it can be a relief and a release to find my own seriousness funny
Accepting – present realities, my own state of mind and it takes time
Decluttering - tidy up, clear out, clean up, mend or throw away
Sustaining hope – believing it will pass; it has been and will be good
Adventuring – experiencing the world as much bigger than my own horizons
Creatureliness – being with, absorbed in and part of nature

References

Adichie, C. (2009) *The danger of a single story* http://www.ted.com/talks/lang/eng/chimamanda_adichie_the_danger_of_a_single_story.html (accessed June 11th 2010)

Bennet, G. (1987) *The Wound and the Doctor: Healing, technology and power in modern medicine.* London: Secker and Warburg.

Braken, P., Thomas, P. (2005) *Postpsychiatry: Mental health in a postmodern world.* Oxford: Oxford University Press.

Coleman, R., Baker, P., Taylor, K. (2000) *Victim to Victor: working to recovery.* Gloucester: Hansell.

Cook, C., Powell, A., Sims., A.(2009) *Spirituality and Psychiatry.* London: Royal College of Psychiatry Publications.

CSIP, RCPsych, SCIE. (2006) *Joint position statement. A common purpose: recovery in future mental health services.* London: Social Care Institute for Excellence. http://www.scie.org.uk/publications/positionpapers/pp08.pdf

Davidson, L., Rakfeldt, J., Strauss, J. (2010) *The Roots of the Recovery Movement in Psychiatry: lessons learned.* Chichester: Wiley.

Daneault, S. (2008) The wounded healer: can this idea be of use to family physicians? *Canadian Family Physician*, 54, 9, 1218-1219 http://www.ncbi. nlm.nih.gov/pmc/articles/PMC2553448/

Estes, C. P. (1992) The ugly duckling: finding what we belong to. Chapter 6 in *Women Who Run with Wolves*. London: Random House.

General Medical Council (2010) *Good medical practice: duties of a doctor.*

Greenhalgh, T., Hurwitz, B. (1998) *Narrative Based Medicine*. London: BMJ Books.

Hunter, K. M. (1991) *Doctors' Stories: the narrative structure of medical knowledge*. Princetown, New Jersey: Princetown University Press.

Klienman, A. (1988) *The Illness Narratives: Suffering, healing and the human condition*. New York: Basic Books.

Leibrich, J. (1999) *A Gift of Stories: discovering how to deal with mental illness*. Dunedin: University of Otago Press

Rakfeldt, J., Strauss, J.S. (1989) The low turning point. A control mechanism in the course of mental disorder. *Journal of Nervous and Mental Disorder*, 177, 1, 32-7.

Rippere, V., Williams, R. (1985) *Wounded Healers: mental health workers experiences of depression*. Chichester: Wiley.

Roberts, G. (1997) Prevention of burnout. *Advances in Psychiatric Treatment*, 3, 5, 282-289.

Roberts, G., & Holmes, J. (1999) *Healing Stories: Narrative in psychiatry and psychotherapy*. Oxford: Oxford University Press

Roberts, G., Davenport, S., Holloway, F., Tattan, T. (2006) *Enabling Recovery: The principles and practice of rehabilitation psychiatry*. London: Gaskell.

Roberts, G., Somers, J., Dawe, J., Passy, R., Mays, C., Carr, G., Shiers, D., Smith, J. (2007) On the Edge: a drama-based mental health education programme on early psychosis for schools. *Early Intervention in Psychiatry*, 1: 168–176

Roberts, G. (1999b) A story of stories. Ch 1 in *Healing Stories: narrative in psychiatry and psychotherapy*, edited by Glenn Roberts and Jeremy Holmes. Oxford: Oxford University Press.

Roberts, G. (2000) Narrative and severe mental illness: what place do stories have in an evidence based world? *Advances in Psychiatric Treatment*, 6, 432-441.

Roberts, G. (2008) e-interview. Psychiatric Bulletin. 32, 80.

Roberts, G. (2009) Coming Home. In *'Beyond the Storms': reflections on personal recovery in Devon*. Edited by Laurie Davidson and Linden Lynn, Devon: Devon Partnership NHS Trust.

Roberts, G., Good, J., Wooldridge, J., Baker, E. (2011) Steps towards, 'Putting recovery at the heart of all we do': workforce development and the role of personal experience. *Journal of Mental Health Training Education and Practice*.

Samuel, R., Thompson, P. (1990) *The Myths We Live By*. London: Routledge.

Shepherd, G., Boardman, J., Burns, M. (2010) *Implementing Recovery: a methodology for organisational change*. London: Sainsbury Centre for Mental Health.

Shepherd, G. Boardman, J. and Slade, M. (2008) *Making Recovery a Reality*. London: Sainsbury Centre for Mental Health.

Strauss, J. (1994) The person with schizophrenia as a person II: approaches to the subjective and complex. *British Journal of Psychiatry*, 164 (suppl. 23), 103-107.

Styron, W. (1991) *Darkness Visible*. London: Picador.

Taylor, D. (1996) *The Healing Power of Stories*. Dublin: Gill and MacMillan.

White, M., Epston, D. (1990) *Narrative Means to Therapeutic Ends*. London: W.W.Norton and Company.

More about Chiron

http://www.youtube.com/watch?v=orxEawi9qro
http://en.wikipedia.org/wiki/Chiron

14
Conclusions:
One man's journey of recovery, is everyone's journey?

Gordon McManus and Jerome Carson

Final reflections

In this concluding chapter, we start by reflecting on the contributions from part 2 of the book, 'Roads to Recovery.' We end with our individual comments on Gordon's own journey, which tie together our thoughts on Part 1 of the book, 'One Man's Long March to Recovery.'

In Chapter 7, Jerome pointed out that recovery is still a comparatively new approach in contemporary mental health services, even though people like Patricia Deegan have been talking about it since the late 1980s. A recent review by the authors Carson, McManus and Chander, (2010), showed that many of the papers, books and policy documents on recovery, have been published in the last few years. The chapter presented a number of local recovery initiatives from the Lambeth South-West Sector. It showed that even small local 'bottom-up' approaches require considerable commitment and resources, from service users and colleagues as well as managerial support and financial assistance.

In Chapter 8, Dr Peter Chadwick, shared his own story of recovery from psychosis. While his story shows that 'you can be induced to madness by being a member of an abused stigmatised minority group,' he goes on to point out that it is possible to 'put it all behind you and move on.' He described how he felt persecuted by his upbringing in the North of England just after the end of World War Two. For him his journey from insanity to recovery was about 'a journey to become who I really am.' The key ingredients of his own recovery were found in love and acceptance and dealing with 'mind healing' as opposed to 'mind wrecking' people. He advised that individuals have to reconstruct a personal narrative through life – and not, as some psychologists might have you believe, via the consulting room. Echoing Rachel Perkins (2011), having a job, accommodation and money, JAM as Peter put it, was vital to rebuilding his life. He focussed his own life on 'meaningfulness and self-realisation,' and to some extent, like Gordon, he also wrote himself well. He ended by saying that 'now the war in his life and head is over,' and he has found 'the peacefulness of a rather Teddy Bear personality.'

Peter started his second chapter, Chapter 9, by looking at the economic costs of schizophrenia. His aim in the chapter, was to ask the question, does having a psychotic episode ever do any good? He suggested that the recent narratives in Cordle et al (2011), present the experiences of people who have had psychosis in a more positive light. He argued that if we focus on individuals' positive qualities, this is both empowering to them and 'hope giving.' Although some people have even stated that being psychotic means you reach a higher level of consciousness, Peter cautioned that, 'Travellers into altered states seek a holiday for the mind but go with no guarantees or insurance.' Jerome once asked Peter what percentage of people who experienced psychosis, would he feel benefitted positively from the experience? His answer was only about 8% of sufferers. Those 8% can however provide inspiring role models for the others.

In Chapter 10, Dolly Sen once more revealed herself to write some of the most evocative and beautiful prose about recovery. In her note to professionals at the start of the chapter, she stated, 'Maybe you will only be the painter of signposts, but to help somebody on the way back to their heart, is the way to go to yours.' She then switched to the nightmare image of her poised above her sleeping father on the verge of stabbing him to death for all the years of abuse she suffered at his hands. It was she says 'the worst point of my life,' and yet it proved to be the beginning of her recovery. She outlined the factors that led to her turning her life around. She provided a list of 27 tips that helped 'propel her life forward.'

In Chapter 11, Dr Duncan Harding and Dr Frank Holloway, explained the significance of nomothetic and idiographic approaches to *Recovery*. While modern evidence based medicine favours nomothetic approaches, they pointed out that people working in mental health services needed 'a profound interest in the individual, their unique personal history and social context.' They highlighted the fact that a lot of the research within the nomothetic tradition was, 'recovery-as-getting-better' and within the idiographic tradition as 'recovery as a journey of the heart.' They also suggested a third strand existed, based on the rights of people with mental health problems to social inclusion and self-determination. They commented that

...*Recovery* is enabled by a transfer of power back to the patient, who should of course be given all the benefits that healthcare can offer but in a manner that is experienced as empowering in order to give them the tools to fashion their own *Recovery*.

They saw a problem with the delivery of *Recovery* oriented care, which might get lost between rhetoric and practice, especially in current services that may be facing extra budgetary pressures.

In Chapter 12, Dr Rachel Perkins told us that she had been working in mental health services for a decade, before she was diagnosed with mental problems herself. Rachel was able to return to her job, despite as she stated, 'having a recurrent mental health problem that takes me back to a psychiatric ward every couple of years or so.' This experience consolidated her belief in trying to ensure that people with psychiatric disabilities would enjoy the same choices she had. Citing Dr Peter Chadwick, Rachel suggested that many professionals were overly focussed on a literature of 'risk, deficit and dysfunction.' Rachel pointed out that 'Employment is ... probably the most important, socially valued and validated way in which we contribute to our communities.' She argued that it was not mental illness per se that stopped people contributing via work, but '... a vicious cycle of low expectations and failure to provide the support and adjustments needed.' In Rachel's view, employment is probably the best route to recovery.

Dr Glenn Roberts wrote about the importance of stories in Chapter 13, and the need for us all '... to find a healing story ... a way of thinking and speaking about our lives, which holds together our truths, our fractured selves, and enables us to become useful, hopeful and helpful to others.' Like others, he too commented that 'Scientific medicine and psychiatry has ... been little interested in stories and seen them as impediments to understanding...' Glenn argued that the recovery movement has chiefly been 'fuelled' by the personal testimony of individuals in recovery. He offered two particular stories in this chapter. For the first, Glenn took us deep into the history of medicine and back to Greek Mythology and Chiron the Centaur. He commented,

Some stories say he (Chiron) invented medicine in an attempt to heal himself but his wound was such that it would not heal and as an immortal he could not die and thus he became both the master of medicine and the original wounded healer ...

The second story was Glenn's own narrative. Following the break-up of his marriage he told us, 'It took about two years before I properly emerged from that depression.' He went onto say, 'I sat so still that for the first time in 25 years my self-winding watch stopped.' Yet this period of dark depression turned out to be a 'low turning point,' as was meeting his second wife, '...the only person I've been comfortable to spend unending time with.' His own experiences of recovering from episodes of depression, have no doubt helped Glenn become the leading British psychiatrist in the recovery field.

Jerome's final thoughts

This book has been constructed around one man's journey of recovery from schizophrenia. As Gordon points out below, it is a journey that is still ongoing. Gordon's family have been with him throughout this journey, especially his mother and sisters, Laura, Gloria and Moira. The dominoes crew of Karl, Stanton, Keith and previously Simmo, have always accepted Gordon, despite his obvious eccentricities during his days at The Studio, when he was floridly mentally ill. They were not aware that he was battling against a severe mental illness at the time. Eric was the son of one of Gordon's best friends, who became a lifelong friend to Gordon. Eric is one of the few people who has seen Gordon in all his 'seasons.' Mental health professionals sometimes refer to such groupings of family and friends, as the patient's 'informal social network.' Yet, these are the people who will always be there for individuals, long after the professionals have gone. Indeed, family and friends may well be the most important people in facilitating recovery.

Gordon is also appreciative of the range and quality of professional support that has been available to him. It was Dr Bindman who gave him a definitive diagnosis. It was also Dr Bindman who wrote to the Courts imploring that Gordon should not be evicted from his flat. Charlene DeVilliers, his social worker and also his care co-ordinator, helped re-establish Gordon back on benefits, and also arranged for his flat to be redecorated. This intervention was equally lifesaving and as Gordon states, he is indebted to Charlene for this. Gordon has also been supported by a range of community psychiatric nurses (CPNs), and both Daisy Masona and Claudette Miller pay tribute to his perseverance and inspiration in dealing with his problems. Several other CPNs have helped along the way including Nadir Mothojokan, Simon Gent and most recently Stellamaris

Adeola, with Dr Indrani Pathmanathan in the 380 medication clinic. It was the late, and much missed, Dr Stephen McGowan, who arranged for Gordon to have CBT at the Maudsley Hospital. This helped accelerate his progress along the recovery care pathway.

It fell to me to try and help Gordon, 'further along the road less travelled.' We developed a five stage model of his recovery together and as he points out, he is at stage 4, 'the stage of recovery.' Stage 5, return to 'a normal life,' remains, at the point of writing, elusive. Will Gordon ever get there? One of his biggest regrets, was his lost years to schizophrenia. Yet, the last four and a half years have seen Gordon not just battle to cope with his own illness, but have seen him come out and share his story with others. His first presentation to our local Recovery Group in February 2008, was a key turning point. He followed this by writing about his experiences and agreeing to appear in Michelle McNary's Recovery Film.

Is Gordon's journey of recovery, everyone's journey? Many writers on the topic of recovery, stress the uniqueness of every individual's journey of recovery (Deegan, 1996). Yet Gordon has faced many of the same difficulties that most sufferers face. He has had to cope with his illness, which has led to four hospital admissions, and he has had to try and find some meaning in his life's journey. For many years Gordon believed that his contributions to communism and the political struggles in Ireland, South Africa and Palestine, gave his life meaning. Mental illness took him away from his dream of being a communist revolutionary. And yet it was mental illness that roused him to wage his greatest battle. In the process I believe that Gordon has become a mental health revolutionary. We need many more brave people like Gordon to come forward and show others that recovery from mental illness is possible. In that sense, Gordon' journey, is the journey that everyone else has to follow. It is as he says, undoubtedly hard work.

Gordon's final thoughts

It is difficult for me to write my section of the Conclusion as I have not recovered from paranoid schizophrenia. As Matt Ward said, in his recovery presentation, it is 'A Work in Progress'.

My recovery stage began after coming out of hospital in 2001 having being diagnosed with paranoid schizophrenia by Dr Bindman. I thank Dr Bindman for the medical care he administered and saving me from being evicted from my flat by Lambeth Council. I thank Charlene for her work. I have never had a better social worker. Most of the time, I did not know where I was during that period of breakdowns. I thank all the nurses and social workers who have looked after me, especially Simon Gent whose intervention led to this collaboration with Dr Carson. Special thanks must go to the late Dr Stephen McGowan who introduced me to therapy.

The most important aspect of my four and a half years of therapy with Dr Carson was the formulation of the 'McManus/Carson model of Recovery'. It provided the clarity that I needed to see how my life had developed over the last thirty years. The model showed that I am in 'the recovery stage' and that I was able to cite Patricia Deegan's definition in my recovery process. I had great difficulties initially in understanding Deegan's definition. This model showed that my goal is full recovery and normal life. This is very important for me and I thank Dr Carson for helping me to structure the model. Without his aid I would have had difficulties.

The recovery stage necessitates a change in attitude as Deegan points out. It entails being open with medical health practitioners so as to get the best from therapy. Therapy has been a 'God-send' (I am an atheist but this is the most apt phrase). It means that I am able to explain my symptoms to another human being who I hope understands. Hope is very important in shaping my attitude in the recovery stage to combat my symptoms. It was Dr Carson who made me aware of hope through giving me articles to read by Deegan and Rachel Perkins. The other qualities needed in the recovery stage from my experience are resolve and determination as Dolly has shown, and perseverance and hard work as Dr Roberts has pointed out. To put it another way 'you have to keep at it', that is, recovery. The mental health service user at the recovery stage cannot allow the symptoms to dominate and control, even though this is difficult. Coping with your symptoms is very important. As Patricia Deegan points out, recovery is not a cure. Writing my chapters meant that I had to confront my life, my mental illness. I had to adopt a new attitude. I had to look at my personality and identity and be aware of my relationships with my family and friends. These are aspects of recovery that Dr Carson made me aware of. It leads to a more meaningful life. The other thing is that when you suffer from mental illness your self-esteem is low and this has to be worked on in the recovery stage. The most important thing for me is to have goals. Through your goals you can work to improve yourself. It is 'hard work' as Dr Roberts has stated.

The experiences of other service users have been invaluable. It provides a 'light' to your own recovery. The 'idiographic' approach is developing and this book in that sense is a contribution. I would like to thank Dolly

Sen, Dr Rachel Perkins, Dr Chadwick and Dr Glenn Roberts for their contributions which have helped me in coping with my symptoms. There are many others. I have mentioned Matt Ward but there is Margaret Muir, Jane Fradgley, Esther Maxwell-Orumbie and those from 380 Streatham High Road, the South-West Community Mental Health Team, who have helped shape my recovery.

The Recovery approach of mental health treatment and the Recovery Movement is now developing in Britain. The contributors in this volume have greatly contributed to that development. I thank them for it because it enhanced my treatment, my Recovery.

The Recovery approach from my experience in the last few years gave me an 'awareness,' as Andresen argues. It entails a new approach to mental health treatment. Something I had not known as I was only used to the medical model. There has to be dialectic between the medical model and the Recovery approach. It entails a 'paradigm shift' about which I hope Dr Carson and I will write an article in the future.

Finally, in my recovery stage there is the domino crew – Stanton Delgado (DJ Stan da Man), Delroy Simpson (Simmo), my domino partner Keith Bent, who bears my anger, and Karl Miller, for treating me as a normal human without stigma and encouraging me. I owe a lot to Eric Ayalande Johnson who has stood by me and keeps a careful watch on me even today.

Dr Carson has 'taught' me that gratitude is very important in mental health recovery. It is with gratitude in mind that I thank the British people for looking after me these last twenty years in my period of mental illness.

I have stated that the goal of full recovery and normal life is very important to me. I have not achieved it yet. Dr Carson and I have discussed that I might not fully recover and that I have to learn to live with schizophrenia towards the end of my therapy with him. Recovery can be both despair and depression at times because of the symptoms and periods of elation when things are going good, that is, life being meaningful. Nevertheless, I shall soldier on to fulfil my goal, the goal of my Individual Recovery Plan or model. It has been and is a 'long march'.

Gordon McManus and Jerome Carson
October 2011
London

References

Carson, J. McManus, G. & Chander, A. (2010) Recovery: a selective review of the literature and resources. *Mental Health and Social Inclusion*, 14, 1, 35-44.

Cordle, H. Fradgley, J. Carson, J. Holloway, F. & Richards, P. (Eds) (2011) *Psychosis Stories of Recovery and Hope*. London: Quay Books.

Deegan, P. (1996) Recovery as a journey of the heart. *Psychiatric Rehabilitation Journal*, 19, 3, 91-97.

Perkins, R. (2011) Rachel Perkins. In, Davies, S. Wakely, E. Morgan, S. & Carson, J. (Eds), *Mental Health Recovery Heroes Past and Present*. Brighton: OLM-Pavilion.

Lightning Source UK Ltd.
Milton Keynes UK
UKOW05f1951050615

252982UK00003B/141/P